T0348632

Avascular Necrosis of the Foot and Ankle

Editor

KENNETH J. HUNT

FOOT AND ANKLE CLINICS

www.foot.theclinics.com

Consulting Editor
MARK S. MYERSON

March 2019 • Volume 24 • Number 1

ELSEVIER

1600 John F. Kennedy Boulevard • Suite 1800 • Philadelphia, Pennsylvania, 19103-2899

http://www.theclinics.com

FOOT AND ANKLE CLINICS Volume 24, Number 1
March 2019 ISSN 1083-7515, ISBN-978-0-323-66104-1

Editor: Lauren Boyle
Developmental Editor: Meredith Madeira

Foot and Ankle Clinics (ISSN 1083-7515) is published quarterly by Elsevier, Inc., 360 Park Avenue South, New York, NY 10010-1710. Months of issue are March, June, September, and December. Periodicals postage paid at New York, NY, and additional mailing offices. Subscription price per year is $337.00 (US individuals), $552.00 (US institutions), $100.00 (US students), $371.00 (Canadian individuals), $663.00 (Canadian institutions), $215.00 (Canadian students), $465.00 (international individuals), $663.00 (international institutions), and $215.00 (international students). To receive student/resident rate, orders must be accompanied by name of affiliated institution, date of term, and the *signature* of program/residency coordinator on institution letterhead. Orders will be billed at individual rate until proof of status is received. Foreign air speed delivery is included in all *Clinics* subscription prices. All prices are subject to change without notice. **POSTMASTER:** Send address changes to *Foot and Ankle Clinics*, Elsevier Health Sciences Division, Subscription Customer Service, 3251 Riverport Lane, Maryland Heights, MO 63043. **Customer Service: 1-800-654-2452 (US and Canada). From outside of the United States and Canada, call 314-447-8871. Fax: 314-447-8029. E-mail: JournalsCustomerService-usa@elsevier.com (for print support); JournalsOnlineSupport-usa@elsevier.com (for online support).**

Reprints. For copies of 100 or more, of articles in this publication, please contact the Commercial Reprints Department, Elsevier Inc., 360 Park Avenue South, New York, NY 10010-1710. Tel.: 212-633-3874; Fax: 212-633-3820; E-mail: reprints@elsevier.com.

Editorial Advisory Board

Contributors

CONSULTING EDITOR

MARK S. MYERSON, MD
Medical Director, The Foot and Ankle Association, Inc, Baltimore, Maryland, USA

EDITOR

KENNETH J. HUNT, MD
Associate Professor and Chief of Foot and Ankle, Department of Orthopaedic Surgery, University of Colorado School of Medicine, Aurora, Colorado, USA

AUTHORS

SAMUEL B. ADAMS, MD
Assistant Professor, Department of Orthopaedic Surgery, Duke University, Durham, North Carolina, USA

JONATHON D. BACKUS, MD
Foot and Ankle Orthopedist, Cornerstone Orthopaedics and Sports Medicine, Superior, Colorado, USA

KIMBERLY BARTOSIAK, MD
Washington University Orthopedics, Washington University School of Medicine in St. Louis, St Louis, Missouri, USA

JEREMY Y. CHAN, MD
Clinical Assistant Professor, Department of Orthopaedics, Stanford University, Stanford, California, USA

MICHAEL P. CLARE, MD
Director, Foot and Ankle Fellowship, Florida Orthopaedic Institute, Tampa, Florida, USA

ELIZABETH A. CODY, MD
Orthopaedic Foot and Ankle Fellow, Duke University Medical Center, Durham, North Carolina, USA

SPENCER COUTURIER, MD, BS
Resident Physician, Department of Radiology, Stanford University, Stanford, California, USA

GARRY GOLD, MD
Professor, Radiology and (by Courtesy) Orthopedics and Bioengineering, Vice Chair for Research, Department of Radiology, Stanford University, Stanford, California, USA

THOMAS G. HARRIS, MD
Chief, Foot and Ankle Surgery, Harbor-UCLA Medical Center, Torrance, California, USA; Foot and Ankle Department, Congress Medical Associates, Pasadena, California, USA

ANDREW HASKELL, MD
Department Lead and Medical Director for Surgical Services, Departments of Orthopedic Surgery and Sports Medicine, Palo Alto Medical Foundation, San Carlos, California, USA

ANGELA K. HEINEN, DO
Fellow, Foot and Ankle Surgery, Harbor-UCLA Medical Center, Torrance, California, USA

JAMES R. LACHMAN, MD
Orthopaedic Foot and Ankle Fellow, Department of Orthopaedic Surgery, Duke University, Durham, North Carolina, USA

ROBERT LELAND, MD
Clinical Assistant Professor, Department of Orthopedic Surgery, University of Colorado School of Medicine, Aurora, Colorado, USA

ERNESTO MACEIRA, MD
Orthopaedic and Trauma Department, Complejo Hospitalario La Mancha Centro, Alcázar de San Juan, Ciudad Real, Spain

PATRICK J. MALONEY, MD
The Institute for Foot and Ankle Reconstruction at Mercy, Baltimore, Maryland, USA

JEREMY J. McCORMICK, MD
Associate Professor of Orthopedic Surgery, Washington University Orthopedics, Washington University School of Medicine in St. Louis, St Louis, Missouri, USA

MICHAEL A. MONT, MD
System Chief of Joint Reconstruction, Vice President, Strategic Initiatives, Lenox Hill Hospital, Northwell Health, New York, New York, USA; Adjunct Staff, Department of Orthopaedic Surgery, Cleveland Clinic, Cleveland, Ohio, USA

MANUEL MONTEAGUDO, MD
Orthopaedic Foot and Ankle Unit, Orthopaedic and Trauma Department, Hospital Universitario Quirónsalud Madrid, Faculty Medicine, UEM Madrid, Madrid, Spain

DANIEL K. MOON, MD, MS, MBA
Assistant Professor, Department of Orthopedic Surgery, University of Colorado School of Medicine, Aurora, Colorado, USA

JAMES A. NUNLEY, MD
Goldner Jones Professor, Department of Orthopaedic Surgery, Duke University Medical Center, Durham, North Carolina, USA

DANIEL L. OCEL, MD
Foot and Ankle Orthopedist, Cornerstone Orthopaedics and Sports Medicine, Superior, Colorado, USA

ASSEM A. SULTAN, MD
Clinical Fellow, Department of Orthopaedic Surgery, Cleveland Clinic, Cleveland, Ohio, USA

YASUHITO TANAKA, MD, PhD
Professor, Chair, Department of Orthopaedic Surgery, Nara Medical University, Kashihara, Nara, Japan

AKIRA TANIGUCHI, MD, PhD
Associate Professor, Department of Orthopaedic Surgery, Nara Medical University, Kashihara, Nara, Japan

ANDREW WAX, BS
Boulder Centre for Orthopedics, Boulder, Colorado, USA

JEFFREY L. YOUNG, MD
Orthopaedic Surgery Resident, Department of Orthopaedics, Stanford University, Stanford, California, USA

Contents

Osteonecrosis arises throughout the foot and ankle in various forms and due to numerous causes, with a thousand US cases per year estimated for the ankle alone. Although research continues to elucidate specific mechanisms at work, the pathophysiology remains poorly understood. Nevertheless, the various osteonecrosis pathways converge on osteocyte death, and bony lesions follow a pattern of progression. Understanding the specific anatomy and biomechanics associated with common forms of foot and ankle osteonecrosis should help guide diagnosis and interventions, particularly at earlier stages of disease where etiology-specific approaches might become optimal.

Avascular necrosis of the foot and ankle is a rare but important cause of pain and functional abnormality. This process may occur in any bone in the foot and ankle; however, it presents most often in characteristic locations. Understanding of key radiographic findings is important in management of these lesions. MRI is the most sensitive and specific method for detection and characterization of this abnormality.

Avascular necrosis (AVN) of the talus bone is a progressive and debilitating consequence of trauma or exposure to a variety of risk factors. The Ficat classification describes current understanding of the natural history of AVN, including preclinical, preradiographic, precollapse, postcollapse, and arthritic stages. The size and location of the avascular region likely determines risk of progression; however, symptoms do not correlate with stage. Patients may be minimally symptomatic despite diffuse involvement for long periods. Joint-sparing strategies have shown promise but do not universally prevent progression of the disease. When bone structure fails, joint-sacrificing strategies may be required.

Displaced talar neck fractures no longer constitute a surgical emergency; timing of definitive surgery has no bearing on the risk of osteonecrosis. Amount of initial fracture displacement is best predictor of osteonecrosis.

Grossly displaced fractures or fracture-dislocations should be provisionally reduced, with or without temporary external fixation. Periosteal stripping should be limited to only that necessary to obtain anatomic reduction. Dissection within the sinus tarsi or tarsal canal should be avoided. Rigid internal fixation with solid cortical screws countersunk within the talar head and placed below the "equator" of the talar head is imperative for optimum stability.

treatment with the use of rigid insoles with medial arch support and a lateral heel wedge is effective in most patients. Dwyer calcaneal osteotomy combined with lateral displacement seems to be a satisfactory treatment for patients who had failed to respond to conservative measures and a good alternative to the different types of perinavicular fusions.

Several operative treatments have been explored to treat patients with progressive or symptomatic osteonecrosis of the talus, aiming to alleviate pain and restore mobility. Because most affected patients are typically younger and more active individuals, joint preservation techniques have received increasing attention. Core decompression, either through an open or percutaneous drilling approach has been used. Similarly, nonvascularized and vascularized bone grafts have been used in clinical practice with varying results. Owing to the relative paucity of studies, in this review we aimed to investigate the use of (1) core decompression and (2) bone grafting for treating osteonecrosis of the talus.

Avascular necrosis (AVN) following rotational ankle fractures is most commonly described in the talus; however, it can also occur in the tibial plafond. These sequelae of ankle fractures are rarely described in the literature. Diagnosis of AVN is best confirmed with MRI of the involved extremity. Treatment options range from conservative treatments such as observation and limited weight-bearing to surgical management including percutaneous drilling, ankle arthrodesis, and total ankle arthroplasty. More research is needed to further identify patients at high risk for developing these sequelae of ankle fractures and to aid in the treatment and surgical decision-making process.

Vascularized bone grafting for talar avascular osteonecrosis is indicated for patients with modified Ficat and Arlet stage I to III disease with minimal subchondral collapse. Outcomes may be more durable than core decompression alone, especially in patients with more advanced disease. Our preferred method, described in this article, involves core decompression followed by use of a vascularized cuboid pedicle graft placed in the defect. Outcomes reported in a small case series have been encouraging, with more than 80% of patients requiring no further surgery.

This article reviews the surgical treatment of talar avascular necrosis. Specifically, arthrodesis for this complex entity and potential treatment of nonunions are discussed. The hallmarks of treatment are evolving and can range from nonoperative measures to amputations. Nonoperative treatment and the results of current arthrodesis techniques for late-stage avascular necrosis are reviewed. Surgical correction requires an understanding of the condition's natural history, utilization of structural and nonstructural bone grafting techniques, and stable fixation. Although the methods described follow standard orthopedic principles, high-quality evidence and outcome studies are limited for treatment of this challenging and often disabling condition.

Severe talar avascular necrosis has many etiologies and can cause bone loss/hindfoot deformity. Tibiotalar calcaneal arthrodesis is a salvage procedure after severe talar avascular necrosis. Large bone voids can present significant challenges. Modest successes have been reported with structural block allograft tibiotalocalcaneal arthrodesis using either plate and screws, intramedullary nail fixation, or a combination. The advent of 3-dimensional printed titanium trusses has given surgeons another option for filling voids and providing structural support to prevent collapse. Although these options expand the armamentarium, treating surgeons must adhere to principles of arthrodesis: stable constructs, thorough joint surface preparation, and correction of deformity.

Avascular necrosis tends to occur in the talus because of poor blood supply caused by the extended coverage to the articular cartilage on its surface. Treatment is conservative in the earlier stage of this disease; however, surgical treatment is usually indicated in the advanced stage. Nonunion, leg length discrepancy, or hindfoot instability may occur in patients treated with ankle or tibio-talo-calcaneal fusion. Arthroplasty using a customized total talar prosthesis designed using the computed tomography image of contralateral talus has the potential advantages of weightbearing in the earlier postoperative phase, prevention of lower extremity discrepancy, and maintenance of joint function.

FOOT AND ANKLE CLINICS

RELATED INTEREST

Orthopedic Clinics, July 2017 (Vol. 48, No. 3)
Orthobiologics
Frederick M. Azar, *Editor*
https://www.orthopedic.theclinics.com

THE CLINICS ARE NOW AVAILABLE ONLINE!
Access your subscription at:
www.theclinics.com

Preface

Management of Avascular Necrosis in the Foot and Ankle

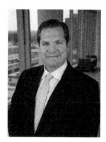

Kenneth J. Hunt, MD
Editor

Avascular necrosis (AVN) involving the bones of the foot and ankle represents a uniquely challenging group of conditions for the foot and ankle surgeon. These rare ailments can strike from a multitude of etiologic pathways and present with a broad range of symptoms and severities. While neither as common nor as easily recognizable as posttraumatic arthritis and lower leg deformity, AVN of bone can lead to considerable disability and compromised function. This makes both recognition and treatment of AVN a challenge for the foot and ankle specialist and underscores the importance of accurately identifying, classifying, and managing these injuries.

Since the early descriptions of AVN conditions by Keonig, there has been significant advancement in our understanding of AVN's causes, diagnostic imaging, medical management of disease, and surgical treatments. Conditions that may have once resulted in severe disability and/or highly invasive and debilitating surgical procedures can often now be managed with progressively less invasive joint and limb-preserving procedures. Better recognition, new implants, and biologic solutions have improved healing rates and outcomes. Still, optimal management of AVN of the foot and ankle requires a deep understanding of the disease process, its broad and disparate causes, and diagnostic and management approaches. While uncommon, the disease is certain to be encountered by foot and ankle providers. And, in some cases, to paraphrase a great mentor, it may have seen you more often than you have seen it.

What is lacking today is a sufficient set of resources for the foot and ankle surgeon to guide recognition and evidence-based management of AVN of the foot and ankle. The rare and variable nature of AVN of the foot and ankle contributes to a paucity of high-level clinical outcomes data and management algorithm, and scarce is a singular resource describing each AVN. The objective of this issue of *Foot and Ankle Clinics of North America* is to provide such a resource for the foot and ankle surgeon. The ensuing articles offer a thorough, up-to-date, and evidence-based review of AVN

Foot Ankle Clin N Am 24 (2019) xv–xvi
https://doi.org/10.1016/j.fcl.2018.12.001
1083-7515/19/© 2018 Published by Elsevier Inc.

foot.theclinics.com

conditions of the foot and ankle to empower the foot and ankle surgeon in the management of these patients, optimize patient outcomes, and help direct the advancement of evolving approaches to treatment.

Kenneth J. Hunt, MD
Department of Orthopaedic Surgery
University of Colorado School of Medicine
12631 East 17th Avenue, Room 4508
Aurora, CO 80045, USA

E-mail address:
Kenneth.j.hunt@ucdenver.edu

Epidemiology, Etiology, and Anatomy of Osteonecrosis of the Foot and Ankle

Daniel K. Moon, MD, MS, MBA

KEYWORDS

- Osteonecrosis • Foot • Ankle • Anatomy • Epidemiology • Cause
- Avascular necrosis

KEY POINTS

- Osteonecrosis of the foot and ankle is less common than in the hip but will be seen repeatedly by foot and ankle specialists; therefore, its causes and related anatomy merit study.
- Osteonecrosis has numerous causes with mechanisms that are often poorly understood but converge on a common pathway of osteocyte death and lesion progression.
- Common presentations of osteonecrosis throughout the foot and ankle vary in how vascular anatomy and biomechanics interact to create conditions for osteonecrosis.

Osteonecrosis is a process in which bone becomes devitalized and can progress to degradation and structural collapse. Osteonecrosis is seen in multiple clinical scenarios as part of varied disease processes and in association with certain drugs, environmental factors, and traumas. Although osteonecrosis may be more common in the hip and knee, foot and ankle specialists will undoubtedly encounter osteonecrosis in various stages and locations during their practice. Despite longstanding awareness of osteonecrosis and exploration of treatment strategies, much about the pathogenesis and progression of osteonecrosis remains poorly understood.

EPIDEMIOLOGY

Most of the osteonecrosis literature and reported epidemiologic data pertains to the femoral head. Foot and ankle osteonecrosis occur less frequently, and some estimates based on reported data are presented here.

Many sources citing that approximately 10% of total hip and ankle joint replacements can be attributed to osteonecrosis are based on a single surgeon's comment (without supporting data) that osteonecrosis "probably accounts for over 10 percent

Disclosure Statement: The author has nothing to disclose.
Department of Orthopedic Surgery, University of Colorado, 12631 East 17th Avenue, Mail Stop B202, Room 4602, Aurora, CO 80045, USA
E-mail address: daniel.moon@ucdenver.edu

of the more than 500,000 total joint replacements performed annually in the United States."[1] Decades after this comment was made, the volume of total joint arthroplasties has increased dramatically to more than 1 million performed in the United States in 2010.[2,3] Such an increase in arthroplasty utilization does not necessarily reflect a proportionally increased osteonecrosis burden, so this estimate may be inaccurate. Nevertheless, hip and knee replacements for osteonecrosis are undoubtedly much more common than foot and ankle surgeries for osteonecrosis.

An epidemiologic survey of osteonecrosis presenting to general practitioners in the United Kingdom found that only 3.1% of all osteonecrosis cases involved the foot or ankle, whereas hip cases accounted for 75.9%.[4] The extrapolated rate of atraumatic hip osteonecrosis in that survey comports well with a separate Japanese epidemiologic survey of idiopathic osteonecrosis of the femoral head. Both studies suggest an incidence of approximately 1.7 cases of atraumatic hip osteonecrosis per 100,000 adults.[5] It is likely that the United Kingdom survey underreported cases of potential foot and ankle osteonecrosis owing to limitations of the national coding system used in the survey. For example, the talus was the only foot bone with a specific avascular necrosis code, and no Freiberg infraction or sesamoid codes were included. The survey data and other reports of osteonecrosis involving the hip, knee, shoulder, and ankle suggest that ankle osteonecrosis comprises 3% to 4% of atraumatic osteonecrosis cases. Ankle lesions are often bilateral or concomitant with lesions at the hip or other sites of the body, suggesting that screening of multiple joints may be prudent when evaluating atraumatic osteonecrosis cases.[4,6–12] The ratio of traumatic to atraumatic osteonecrosis cases of the talus have been reported as high as 3 to 1.[6,13]

If these estimates are applied to the US population, at least 250 cases of atraumatic, adult foot and ankle osteonecrosis cases would be expected per year. Thus, including traumatic etiologies, approximately 1000 adult ankle osteonecrosis cases may present annually in the United States. This figure does not include the variety of other potential forefoot and midfoot osteonecrosis patients seen by foot and ankle providers, which would increase the total estimate of annual US foot and ankle osteonecrosis cases even higher.

ETIOLOGY

Osteonecrosis is only 1 of numerous terms used to describe similar pathologic outcomes of bone, such as avascular necrosis, aseptic necrosis, ischemic necrosis, and bone infarction.

The list of conditions (**Box 1**) associated with osteonecrosis is quite long, though not all have been conclusively shown to actually cause osteonecrosis.[14] Even when a causal relationship is present, the mechanisms are often unclear.

Traumatic Osteonecrosis

Osteonecrosis most frequently arises as a consequence of traumatic injuries, and the hip is the most common location; for example, after femoral neck fractures and hip dislocations. In the foot and ankle, traumatic osteonecrosis is most commonly associated with talar fractures. Overall rates of osteonecrosis following talar fractures were reported as high as 58% in the original description by Hawkins[15,16] (42% for Hawkins type II, 86% for type III) and other early reports. However, reported rates of osteonecrosis have decreased over time, particularly for type II and type III fractures, such that overall osteonecrosis rates after talar fractures are now reported at approximately 25% to 30%. These decreased rates are potentially due to advances in treatment and fixation.[17–19]

Box 1
Conditions associated with osteonecrosis

Trauma
  Burns
  Fractures
  Dislocations
  Vascular trauma
  Kienböck disease

Nontraumatic conditions
  Hematologic
    Hemoglobinopathies
      Sickle-cell anemia
      Thalassemias
    Disseminated intravascular coagulation
    Polycythemia
    Hemophilia
  Metabolic or endocrinologic
    Hypercholesterolemia
    Gout
    Hyperparathyroidism
    Hyperlipidemia
    Pregnancy
    Cushing disease
    Chronic renal failure
    Gaucher disease
    Diabetes (in association with obesity)
    Fabry disease
  Gastrointestinal
    Pancreatitis
    Inflammatory bowel disease
  Neoplastic
    Marrow infiltrative disorders
  Infectious
    Osteomyelitis
    Human immunodeficiency virus
    Meningococcemia
  Vascular, rheumatologic, or connective tissue
  Disorders
    Systemic lupus erythematosus
    Polymyositis
    Polymyalgia rheumatica
    Raynaud disease
    Rheumatoid arthritis
    Ankylosing spondylitis
    Sjögren syndrome
    Giant cell arteritis
    Thrombophlebitis
    Lipid emboli
    Ehler-Danlos syndrome
  Orthopedic problems
    Slipped capital femoral epiphysis
    Congenital hip dislocation
    Hereditary dysostosis
    Legg- Calvé-Perthes disease
  Extrinsic dietary or environmental factors
    Dysbaric conditions (Caisson disease)
    Alcohol consumption
    Cigarette smoking

Iatrogenic
  Corticosteroids
  Radiation exposure
  Hemodialysis
  Organ transplantation
  Laser surgery
Idiopathic

From Assouline-Dayan Y, Chang C, Greenspan A, et al. Pathogenesis and natural history of osteonecrosis. Semin Arthritis Rheum 2002;32(2):96, with permission.

In a displaced fracture, nutrient arteries can be disrupted, and associated soft tissue damage may decrease local blood flow. Both the fracture itself and applied fixation may interfere with periosteal blood flow. Early bone porosis underneath implants can result from remodeling induced by a small degree of localized necrosis. In the case of talus fractures, the degree of associated joint subluxation or dislocation at time of injury and the concomitant interruption of limited blood supply vessels seem to be a particularly important factor in the development of osteonecrosis.[20]

Traumatic injuries may exert sufficient influence to cause the development of osteonecrosis independently; however, additional atraumatic risk factors can also compound and magnify the potential for a given traumatic injury to progress to osteonecrosis.[21]

Atraumatic Osteonecrosis

Corticosteroids

Corticosteroid use is the most commonly cited etiology of atraumatic osteonecrosis, and it has multiple adverse effects on bone that ultimately lead to its failure. Interestingly, increasing evidence suggests that the term osteonecrosis may be inaccurate in this case. Corticosteroids induce apoptosis of osteoblasts and osteocytes, and histologic specimens from femoral heads with steroid-associated collapse demonstrate apoptotic osteocytes with condensed nuclei and fragmented chromatin in the lacunae in contrast to the vacant lacunae seen in true osteonecrosis secondary to trauma (**Fig. 1**). Absent the mechanosensory actions of the osteocytes, bone adaptation and remodeling are potentially impaired.[22] Corticosteroids also potentiate osteoclast survival, which combines with their proapoptotic effect on osteoblasts to lead to rapid decreases in bone mineral density, as demonstrated in mice.[23]

There are mechanisms by which glucocorticoids may also promote vascular compromise and ischemic necrosis. Glucocorticoids may interfere directly with angiogenesis and vascular endothelial growth factor (VEGF) production and action.[24] In addition, because osteocytes and osteoblasts promote angiogenesis, their apoptotic losses indirectly diminish vascular growth further.

Another proposed mechanism for osteonecrosis has been marrow fat hypertrophy and hyperplasia in response to glucocorticoids, which increases intracortical pressure and decreases intraosseous blood.[25] However, evidence suggests that this may only play a partial role because osteonecrosis does not necessarily occur with elevated intraosseous pressures.[26] Lipids have been shown to accumulate in human and rabbit osteocytes in the setting of steroids, which is consistent with increased lipids found in osteonecrotic femoral heads. However, it remains unclear whether this increased lipid content directly causes impaired vascularity or osteonecrosis as theorized.[27–29]

A dose-response relationship between steroids and hip osteonecrosis formation has been demonstrated. A meta-analysis demonstrated that exceeding 20 mg per

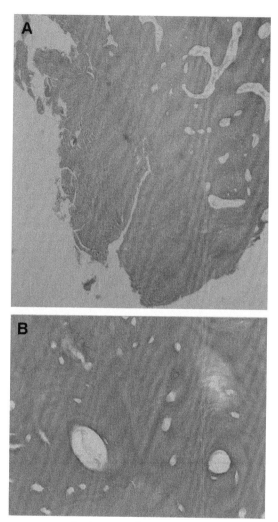

Fig. 1. Histologic appearance of osteonecrosis. Bone and cartilage section from osteonecrotic sesamoid (*A*). Magnification of bone demonstrating empty lacunae devoid of osteocytes (*B*).

day of prednisone-equivalent led to an increased odds ratio for developing osteonecrosis of 9.1 (95% CI 4.6–19.8). Similarly, exceeding 10 g of cumulative dose led to an increased odds ratio of 2.4 (95% CI 0.8–6.4).[30] The risk for developing osteonecrosis of the femoral head seems to be highest during the first few months after initiating corticosteroid treatment; however, the risk period extends until approximately 12 months after initiation.[31,32] These clinical guidelines and risk period may not translate perfectly to foot and ankle osteonecrosis; however, it seems reasonable to limit corticosteroid dosing in general and to monitor for osteonecrosis as an adverse effect for a year after meaningful exposure.

Alcohol
Excessive alcohol use has long been identified as a risk factor for osteonecrosis, though only a small percentage of alcoholics develop osteonecrosis. As with

corticosteroids, multiple mechanisms have been proposed for alcohol-related osteo-necrosis; however, uncertainty remains. Some potential mechanisms being investi-gated for alcohol-related bone dysfunction also overlap with steroid-induced osteonecrosis. Alcohol use has been associated with osteoporosis, and rat studies have shown that alcohol also causes osteocyte apoptosis and lipid proliferation.[33]

Studies have also demonstrated genetic factors associated with osteonecrosis. Aldehyde dehydrogenase 2 (ALDH2) is a key enzyme in alcohol metabolism, for which there is a high prevalence of an inactive allele variant among East Asians that causes flushing and discomfort with drinking but is protective against alcoholism.[34] The 12q24 gene locus containing ALDH2 and the 20q12 locus have been associated with idiopathic and alcohol-induced osteonecrosis of the femoral head in Japanese populations.[35] A specific mechanism by which the acetaldehyde accumulation promotes osteonecrosis is not clear; however, lipid dysfunction is a proposed mechanism.[36,37]

A dose-response relationship between alcohol and osteonecrosis risk has been demonstrated in multiple studies. Risks increase for occasional drinkers (<8 mL per day) and even further for regular drinkers (>8 mL per day).[38,39] A comparative study showed that, although alcohol increases risk for osteonecrosis (11.1 odds ratio for those who do not use steroids; 95% CI 1.3–95.5), corticosteroid-induced risk is much higher (31.5 odds ratio for nondrinkers; 95% CI 9.05–109), to the degree that odds do not change much for drinkers taking corticosteroids, reflecting the over-whelming inherent risk from corticosteroids alone.[40]

Smoking
Smoking increases the risk of osteonecrosis of the femoral head; however, the precise mechanism is unclear.[38,39] Suggested mechanisms include smoking's deleterious effects on nitric oxide bioavailability, increased oxidative stress, and damage to endo-thelium.[41] A dose-response relationship has been demonstrated, though weaker than with alcohol. Nevertheless, osteonecrosis risks seem to be consistently increased for current smokers, smoking more than 20 cigarettes per day, and a history greater than 25 pack-years. Similar to the alcohol findings, the odds ratio increase was less impres-sive for smokers with current or past corticosteroid use than for the corticosteroid-naïve smokers versus nonsmokers.[41]

Sickle cell disease
In sickle cell disease, multiple mechanisms are thought to contribute to osteonecrosis. Abnormal polymerization of hemoglobin and subsequent red cell sickling morphology seem to impair perfusion by increasing blood viscosity, causing stasis, and occluding vessels.[42,43] Subchondral bone infarcts can lead to eventual collapse.[44] Although sickle cell disease is itself a risk factor for osteonecrosis, this risk may be amplified by variation in genes such as annexin A2, bone morphogenetic protein 6, and klotho; which potentially increase vascular inflammation, oxidant stress, and endothelial damage.[45]

A study of osteonecrotic tali in subjects with sickle cell disease demonstrated that talar osteonecrosis, when present, was always concomitant with hip osteonecrosis and never in isolation at the foot and ankle. Subjects with the most severe SS sickle cell genotype were also at highest risk of rapid talus collapse, which followed symp-tom presentation within 5 years. No cases of osteonecrotic lesion regression were seen, and symptomatic lesions progressed to collapse faster than asymptomatic ones. In this group, collapse of the posterior and middle talus was more likely than the anterior portion.[12]

Other risk factors

Among patients taking corticosteroids, those with systemic lupus erythematosus have been shown to be at significantly higher risk for osteonecrosis.[9] After observing a pattern of coagulation dysfunction across a group of osteonecrotic patients with various conditions, an emphasis on procoagulative states has been proposed as a an etiology of osteonecrosis. This state could be due to formal disorders, such as anti-phospholipid syndrome and thrombophilia, but also includes patients with procoagu-lative sequelae of corticosteroid use or alcohol abuse.[46] Studies of antiphospholipid syndrome have been mixed on this mechanism. Some have demonstrated a potential effect on osteonecrosis development beyond corticosteroid use; however, others have not.[7,47–49]

Gaucher disease is associated with osteonecrosis; however, the precise etiology of lesions is unknown. The accumulation of glucocerebrosidase within marrow cells was previously thought to create vascular compression and occlusion, and engorged mac-rophages were theorized to block small vessels. However, histologic evidence sug-gests that bone vessels are devoid of Gaucher cells, and radionuclide trackers suggest blood flow to bone may actually be increased in affected bone and marrow, arguing against vascular insufficiency.[50] Nevertheless, enzymatic treatment of Gaucher disease with recombinant ß-glucocerebrosidase has been shown to decrease bone pain and decrease the rate of osteonecrosis development.[51] This may suggest either a unique or more complex interplay of factors causing osteonec-rosis in Gaucher disease.

Clearly, the causes and risk factors associated with osteonecrosis are legion and variable. There may at times be some overlap among the pathogenic mechanisms of certain diseases, environmental exposures, and traumatic etiologies. At the same time, some causes of osteonecrosis have unique mechanisms. The complexity of po-tential mechanisms suggests that may never be a single, universal intervention to pre-vent osteonecrosis and that optimal approaches to prevention and treatment will be etiology-specific.

Osteonecrosis Lesion Progression

Importantly, there is a distinction between osteonecrosis of bone tissue and the devel-opment of structural deficiencies and failure. Multiple orthopedic classification sys-tems for osteonecrosis note that stages of intrinsic tissue change precede any structural fracture or collapse. For example, stage 1 of the Ficat and Arlet classification (originally for the hip but modified for the talus) is radiographically silent with changes only seen on MRI.[6] Stage 0 of the Steinberg classification system describes a stage of osteonecrosis devoid of both radiographic and MRI changes.[52]

The various causes of osteonecrosis demonstrate that a complex array of factors influence osteocyte viability. However, the various pathways converge on osteocyte death and the potential for later collapse (**Fig. 2**).

Reparative responses in atraumatic and traumatic osteonecrosis may differ with respect to marrow reaction and lamellar versus woven bone formation; however, the general reparative process in both cases is characterized by new appositional, living bone laid on the dead trabeculae in the subchondral bone, as well as resorption of dead trabeculae. Overall, resorption outpaces bone formation, leading to a loss of bone density in areas subject to repair. These areas are susceptible to potential micro-fracture, which can accumulate to the point of prompting subchondral collapse, macroscopic fracture, and joint incongruities. The density of unrepaired dead bone re-mains unchanged. Thus, subchondral fractures and collapse are not the result of oste-ocyte death, per se, but are likely the result of the resorptive component of the

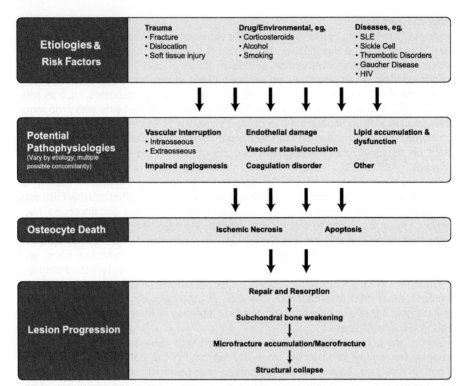

Fig. 2. Osteonecrosis pathophysiology and lesion progression illustrating convergence of multiple etiologic pathways. HIV, human immunodeficiency virus; SLE, systemic lupus erythematosus.

reparative response.[53,54] As stresses are applied to an osteonecrotic bone, the likelihood of structural failure is primarily driven by the accumulated regions of weakened subchondral cancellous bone undermining the joint rather than a deficient subchondral plate itself.[55] The size and locations of weakened subchondral cancellous bone interact to determine the likelihood of macro-level structural collapse.[56]

In general, it does seem that traumatic cases of avascular necrosis demonstrate a more robust tissue reparative response than atraumatic cases.[53] This may explain the proportion of traumatic talar osteonecrosis cases in which revascularization is able to reverse osteonecrosis radiographic findings in the dome without any subsequent bony collapse.[17,53]

ANATOMY

Although osteonecrosis has been reported throughout the entire foot and ankle, some anatomic sites present with greater frequency than others due to their vascular supply and stress-bearing characteristics (**Fig. 3**). Although these specific bones and regions are beyond the scope of this article (see later discussion of the most common sites of osteonecrosis in the foot and ankle).

Talus

With 3 major articulations (tibiotalar, subtalar, and talonavicular) simultaneously transmitting various moments and stresses through the talus, it may not be surprising that

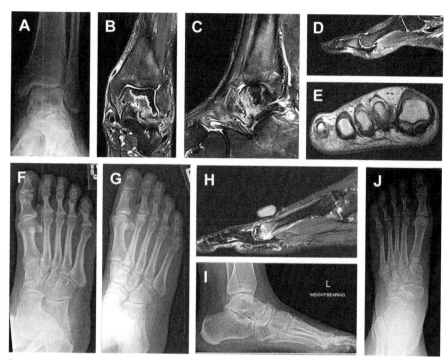

Fig. 3. Radiograph and MRI examples of common forms of foot and ankle osteonecrosis. Posttraumatic talar osteonecrosis (*A–C*). Chronic sesamoid osteonecrosis (*D–F*). Freiberg infraction of second metatarsal (*G, H*). Müller-Weiss (*I, J*).

the talus is a frequent location for osteonecrosis in the foot and ankle. Approximately 60% of the talus surface is covered with cartilage[57] and there are no tendinous nor muscular attachments. With only a minor portion of its surface available for rich periosteal circulation enjoyed by most bone,[21] the talus is vulnerable to vascular disruptions. However, vulnerability should not be confused with poor baseline perfusion. The talus derives its blood supply from branches of 3 major regional vessels: the anterior tibial, posterior tibial, and peroneal arteries. The artery of the tarsal canal is the largest contributor branch, followed by the deltoid and sinus tarsi branches, leaving the superior neck and posterior tubercle vessels as relatively minor sources.[58]

Although both the femoral head and talus are largely covered by cartilage, the low frequency of atraumatic talar osteonecrosis relative to femoral head osteonecrosis might be explained, in part, by the proportionately larger, uninterrupted expanse of the femoral head cartilage versus the discrete patches of articular surface on the talus with 5 interposed areas available for feeder vessels.

The regions of the talus most affected by osteonecrosis seem to depend on the etiology. In traumatic osteonecrosis after talar neck fractures (eg, Hawkins type IIB or III), the anterolateral region of the talar dome seems to be more commonly affected by collapse.[59,60] In talar neck fractures, the intraosseous branches and artery to the tarsal canal are disrupted. With type IIB and III fractures, the deltoid branch of the tibial artery is also likely to be disrupted by the subtalar dislocation, increasing the risk of osteonecrosis.[20] In contrast, atraumatic osteonecrosis can center on the posterolateral region of the talar dome, the region with the poorest baseline vascular supply.[6]

Navicular

Osteonecrosis of the navicular can result after trauma or can develop spontaneously. Navicular fractures have been classified into 3 types: type 1 fractures separate the navicular into dorsal and plantar fragments, type 2 fractures split the navicular along a more sagittal plane from dorsal-lateral to plantar-medial, and type 3 denotes comminution along the sagittal plane often accompanied by loss of medial column height and length. Although type 2 fractures are the most common, osteonecrosis is most associated with types 1 and 3 fracture patterns.[61]

Köhler disease and Müller-Weiss disease are often described as presentations of atraumatic navicular osteonecrosis in children and adults, respectively. Limited reports of histologic samples from Köhler disease patients have described dead trabeculae.[62] However, the radiologic appearance of increased sclerosis and navicular flattening are identical to those found in many asymptomatic patients, and some sources describe Köhler disease as an osteochondrosis process that is distinct from osteonecrosis.[63] Notably, the radiographic navicular abnormalities resolve in both symptomatic and asymptomatic children, irrespective of weight-bearing or immobilization treatment. Thus, it remains unclear whether Köhler disease represents a symptomatic abnormality of ossification that is self-limited after maturation or, alternatively, a truly osteonecrotic process that spontaneously resolves.

In contrast, the adult Müller-Weiss disease patient exhibits a potential for permanent deformity (eg, rearfoot varus) and eccentric collapse of the lateral navicular. Multiple European reports have noted histologic findings in Müller-Weiss disease patients that are inconsistent with osteonecrosis; however, others have reported histologic findings that are consistent with osteonecrosis (eg, empty lacunae).[64–66]

Early descriptions of navicular vascular supply noted a central region of hypovascularity.[67] This watershed region has been considered a factor contributing to the development of osteonecrosis, particularly in posttraumatic cases,[61] as well as potentially influencing stress fracture treatment.[68] More recent work has demonstrated that the presence and location of a hypovascular region is variable among patients. Medial and lateral tarsal branches derived from the dorsalis pedis artery are consistent, as is a branch to the plantar navicular from the medial plantar artery. Frequently, the plantar and medial vessels form an anastomotic ring around the navicular tuberosity. The hypovascular region was central in only 12% of specimens and did not necessarily extend to the dorsal surface. In other patients, the hypovascular region may be more lateral or not even present at all.[69]

It has been theorized that differential stresses between the medial versus middle columns can create a shear stress in the central navicular that influences Müller-Weiss disease and stress fracture development, particularly in the presence of a shortened first ray or long second ray.[64,70] Thus, a combination of structural and vascular anomalies may make some individuals more prone to the formation of navicular osteonecrosis than the broader population; for example, increased central stress or fracture of the navicular in a small percentage of patients with central hypovascularity.

First Metatarsal

Osteonecrosis of the first metatarsal is mostly reported as an iatrogenic consequence of hallux valgus correction and reports of idiopathic necrosis are uncommon.[71,72] Distal osteotomies in conjunction with lateral soft tissue release were reported to have up to a 40% risk of osteonecrosis.[73] Later work demonstrated that radiographic changes potentially consistent with osteonecrosis are present in a small percentage of patients (7%–25%) but that clinical symptoms are uncommon.[74–77]

The first metatarsal head receives extraosseous blood supply from branches off the first dorsal metatarsal artery, the first plantar metatarsal artery, and the medial plantar artery. Branches from these vessels invest into the periosteum, which then sends tiny vessels that penetrate the cortex. Dissections suggest that the vessels form a plexus that is centered on the plantar-lateral aspect of the head, which makes it vulnerable to errant distal osteotomy saw cuts (eg, Chevron) that extend beyond the bone into the soft tissues.[78,79]

Intraosseous flow is augmented by a nutrient vessel that branches off the first dorsal metatarsal artery and consistently enters the lateral first metatarsal, typically in the distal third or at the junction of the distal and middle thirds. After penetrating the cortex, the vessel branches proximally and distally. All distal osteotomies disrupt the intraosseous supply, so the general guidance remains to avoid overstripping the soft tissues surrounding the metatarsal head and to ensure that saw cuts do not damage the vasculature lateral to the first metatarsal.[76,80]

Lesser Metatarsals

Unlike the first metatarsal, reports of iatrogenic osteonecrosis of the lesser metatarsals after surgery are uncommon.[81] Instead, lesser metatarsal osteonecrosis is most commonly seen with spontaneous osteonecrosis of the metatarsal head (typically the second), that is, Freiberg disease or Freiberg infraction.

The lesser metatarsal heads receive blood from branches off the dorsal metatarsal arteries stemming from the dorsalis pedis and from the plantar metatarsal arteries stemming from the posterior tibial artery. These branches form anastomoses around the metatarsal heads, and a nutrient artery typically enters around the ligamentous and capsular origins.[82]

With a reasonable extraosseous and intraosseous supply present, physical stresses or trauma seem to bear more influence on the development of Freiberg disease. The second metatarsal is typically the longest, and its head may experience more stress in weightbearing and toe-off, creating a dorsal-distal lesion on the head. In many cases, hallux valgus deformity causes the transfer of weight away from the first metatarsal to the second, exacerbating the stresses seen.[83,84]

Sesamoids

Case reports of sesamoid osteonecrosis dating back to 1924 first noted the more commonly affected medial sesamoid; however, lateral sesamoids can also be affected.[85–87] Histologic examples have been consistent with osteonecrosis but the exact cause is not clear. The initiating etiology of sesamoid osteonecrosis is thought to be microfractures from repetitive stress or trauma, which eventually interfere with the vascular supply and remodeling.

The vascular supply to the sesamoids is somewhat variable and can originate from the medial plantar artery or the plantar arch. The first plantar metatarsal artery supplies the lateral sesamoid and sometimes also sends branches to the medial sesamoid (proximal, or proximal and distal). In other cases, the medial sesamoid is supplied by the proper plantar artery. Each sesamoid is penetrated by arteries at its proximal, plantar, and distal aspects.[88,89]

Given the anatomic variability of flow, the conditions for developing sesamoid osteonecrosis may depend on an infrequent combination of specific biomechanical stresses or traumatic events and certain vascular anatomy patterns.

SUMMARY

Significant headway is being made with respect to understanding the etiologies and risk factors associated with osteonecrosis, though much remains to be explored. Compared with hip osteonecrosis, symptomatic foot and ankle osteonecrosis occurs far less frequently and with more diverse presentation, which has made dedicated study more difficult. However, knowledge gained from the hip literature may at times be transferable to the foot and ankle. The use of specialty-specific data registries in the future may enable more thorough foot-specific and ankle-specific studies of osteonecrosis because more data from the thousand or more annual cases could be pooled. Although perhaps not an everyday horse, osteonecrosis is also not a zebra for foot and ankle specialists.

The common endpoints of osteocyte death and structural collapse are present along multiple pathways; however, effective intervention at earlier stages is a future challenge. Better understanding of the pathogenesis may create pathway-specific opportunities for reversal, prevention, or less invasive procedures. At the same time, multiple risk factors may overlap in certain patients such that they may be best served by multipronged approaches combining surgical interventions with medical and therapeutic adjuncts. Because osteonecrosis of the foot and ankle has a myriad of presentations and sites, our understanding of the structural, vascular, and biomechanical anatomy of the foot and ankle is critical to the development of optimal treatment strategies for each kind of osteonecrosis seen in our practices' complex assortment of pathologic conditions.

REFERENCES

1. Mankin H. Nontraumatic necrosis of bone (Osteonecrosis). N Eng J Med 1992; 326(22):1473–9.
2. Williams SN, Wolford ML, Bercovitz A. Hospitalization for total knee replacement among inpatients aged 45 and over: United States, 2000-2010. NCHS Data Brief 2015;210:1–8.
3. Wolford ML, Palso K, Bercovitz A. Hospitalization for total hip replacement among inpatients aged 45 and over: United States, 2000-2010. NCHS Data Brief 2015; 186:1–8.
4. Cooper C, Steinbuch M, Stevenson R, et al. The epidemiology of osteonecrosis: findings from the GPRD and THIN databases in the UK. Osteoporos Int 2010; 21(4):569–77.
5. Fukushima W, Fujioka M, Kubo T, et al. Nationwide epidemiologic survey of idiopathic osteonecrosis of the femoral head. Clin Orthop Relat Res 2010;468(10): 2715–24.
6. Delanois RE, Mont MA, Yoon TR, et al. Atraumatic osteonecrosis of the talus. J Bone Joint Surg Am 1998;80-A(4):529–36.
7. Gladman D, Dhillon N, Su J, et al. Osteonecrosis in SLE: prevalence, patterns, outcomes and predictors. Lupus 2018;27:76–81.
8. Issa K, Naziri Q, Kapadia BH, et al. Clinical characteristics of early-stage osteonecrosis of the ankle and treatment outcomes. J Bone Joint Surg Am 2014;96(9):e73.
9. Shigemura T, Nakamura J, Kishida S, et al. Incidence of osteonecrosis associated with corticosteroid therapy among different underlying diseases: prospective MRI study. Rheumatology (Oxford) 2011;50(11):2023–8.
10. Castro TC, Lederman H, Terreri MT, et al. The use of joint-specific and whole-body MRI in osteonecrosis: a study in patients with juvenile systemic lupus erythematosus. Br J Radiol 2011;84(1003):621–8.

11. Chollet CT, Britton L, Neel MD, et al. Childhood cancer survivors. Clin Orthop Relat Res 2005;(430):149–55.
12. Hernigou P, Flouzat-Lachaniette CH, Daltro G, et al. Talar osteonecrosis related to adult sickle cell disease: natural evolution from early to late stages. J Bone Joint Surg Am 2016;98(13):1113–21.
13. Adelaar RS, Madrian JR. Avascular necrosis of the talus. Orthop Clin North Am 2004;35(3):383–95, xi.
14. Assouline-Dayan Y, Chang C, Greenspan A, et al. Pathogenesis and natural history of osteonecrosis. Semin Arthritis Rheum 2002;32(2):94–124.
15. Hawkins LG. Fractures of the neck of the talus. J Bone Joint Surg Am 1970;52:91–1002.
16. Canale ST, Kelly FBJ. Fractures of the neck of the talus. Long-term evaluation of seventy-one cases. J Bone Joint Surg Am 1978;60(2):143–56.
17. Vallier HA, Reichard SG, Boyd AJ, et al. A new look at the Hawkins classification for talar neck fractures: which features of injury and treatment are predictive of osteonecrosis? J Bone Joint Surg Am 2014;96(3):192–7.
18. Dodd A, Lefaivre K. Outcomes of talar neck fractures: a systematic review and meta-analysis. J Orthop Trauma 2015;29(5):210–5.
19. Jordan RK, Bafna KR, Liu J, et al. Complications of talar neck fractures by Hawkins classification: a systematic review. J Foot Ankle Surg 2017;56(4):817–21.
20. Lin SS, Montemurro NJ. New modification to the Hawkins classification scheme is more predictive of osteonecrosis: commentary on an article by Heather A. Vallier, MD, et al.: "A new look at the Hawkins classification for talar neck fractures: which features of injury and treatment are predictive of osteonecrosis?". J Bone Joint Surg Am 2014;96(3):e25.
21. McCarthy I. The physiology of bone blood flow: a review. J Bone Joint Surg Am 2006;88(Suppl 3):4–9.
22. Weinstein RS, Nicholas RW, Manolagas SC. Apoptosis of osteocytes in glucocorticoid-induced osteonecrosis of the hip. J Clin Endocrinol Metab 2000;85(8):2907–12.
23. Jia D, O'Brien CA, Stewart SA, et al. Glucocorticoids act directly on osteoclasts to increase their life-span and reduce bone density. Endocrinology 2006;147(12):5592–9.
24. Weinstein RS, Wan C, Liu Q, et al. Endogenous glucocorticoids decrease angiogenesis, vascularity, hydration, and strength in aged mice. Aging Cell 2010;9:147–61.
25. Wang GJ, Cui Q, Balian G. The pathogenesis and prevention of steroid induced osteonecrosis. Clin Orthop Relat Res 2000;370:295–310.
26. Atsumi T, Kuroki Y. Role of impairment of blood supply of the femoral head in the pathogenesis of idiopathic osteonecrosis. Clin Orthop Relat Res 1992;277:22–30.
27. Kawai K, Tamaki A, Hirohata K. Steroid-induced accumulation of lipid in the osteocytes of the rabbit femoral head. A histochemical and electron microscopic study. J Bone Joint Surg Am 1985;67(5):755–63.
28. Uno K, Kawai K, Hirohata K, et al. Steroid induced early changes of the femoral head in man - histological study of autopsied cases. Ryumachi 1991;31(3):282–9.
29. Boskey AL, Raggio CL, Bullough PG, et al. Changes in the bone tissue lipids in persons with steroid- and alcohol-induced osteonecrosis. Clin Orthop Relat Res 1983;172:289–95.
30. Mont MA, Pivec R, Banerjee S, et al. High-dose corticosteroid use and risk of hip osteonecrosis: meta-analysis and systematic literature review. J Arthroplasty 2015;30(9):1506–12.e5.

31. Sakamoto M, Shimizu K, Ida S, et al. Osteonecrosis of the femoral head. J Bone Joint Surg Br 1997;79-B:213–9.
32. Fink B, Degenhardt S, Paselk C, et al. Early detection of avascular necrosis of the femoral head following renal transplantation. Arch Orthop Trauma Surg 1997;116: 151–6.
33. Maurel DB, Pallu S, Jaffre C, et al. Osteocyte apoptosis and lipid infiltration as mechanisms of alcohol-induced bone loss. Alcohol Alcohol 2012;47(4):413–22.
34. Li H, Borinskaya S, Yoshimura K, et al. Refined geographic distribution of the OrientalALDH2*504Lys(nee487Lys) variant. Ann Hum Genet 2009;73(3):335–45.
35. Sakamoto Y, Yamamoto T, Sugano N, et al. Genome-wide association study of idiopathic osteonecrosis of the femoral head. Sci Rep 2017;7(1):15035.
36. Yoon BH, Kim TY, Shin IS, et al. Alcohol intake and the risk of osteonecrosis of the femoral head in Japanese populations: a dose-response meta-analysis of case-control studies. Clin Rheumatol 2017;36(11):2517–24.
37. Zhang W, Zhong W, Sun X, et al. Visceral white adipose tissue is susceptible to alcohol-induced lipodystrophy in rats: role of acetaldehyde. Alcohol Clin Exp Res 2015;39(3):416–23.
38. Matsuo K, Hirohata T, Sugioka Y, et al. Influence of alcohol intake, cigarette smoking, and occupational status on idiopathic osteonecrosis of the femoral head. Clin Orthop Relat Res 1988;234:115–23.
39. Hirota Y, Hirohata T, Fukuda K, et al. Association of alcohol intake, cigarette smoking, and occupational status with the risk of idiopathic osteonecrosis of the femoral head. Am J Epidemiol 1993;137:530–8.
40. Fukushima W, Yamamoto T, Takahashi S, et al. The effect of alcohol intake and the use of oral corticosteroids on the risk of idiopathic osteonecrosis of the femoral head. Bone Joint J 2013;95(3):320–5.
41. Takahashi S, Fukushima W, Kubo T, et al. Pronounced risk of nontraumatic osteonecrosis of the femoral head among cigarette smokers who have never used oral corticosteroids: a multicenter case-control study in Japan. J Orthop Sci 2012; 17(6):730–6.
42. Diggs LW, Bell A. Intraerythrocyte hemoglobin crystals in sickle cell-hemoglobin C disease. Blood 1965;25(2):218–23.
43. Nascor ZA, Bachabi M, Jones LC, et al. Osteonecrosis in sickle cell disease. South Med J 2016;109(9):525–30.
44. Hernigou P, Habibi A, Bachir D, et al. The natural history of asymptomatic osteonecrosis of the femoral head in adults with sickle cell disease. J Bone Joint Surg Am 2006;88-A(12):2565–72.
45. Baldwin C, Nolan VG, Wyszynski DF, et al. Association of klotho, bone morphogenic protein 6, and annexin A2 polymorphisms with sickle cell osteonecrosis. Blood 2005;106:372–5.
46. Jones LC, Mont MA, Tung BL, et al. Procoagulants and osteonecrosis. J Rheumatol 2003;30:783–91.
47. Vasoo S, Sangle S, Zain M, et al. Orthopaedic manifestations of the antiphospholipid (Hughes) syndrome. Lupus 2005;14:339–45.
48. Zalavras C, Dailiana Z, Elisaf M, et al. Potential aetiological factors concerning the development of osteonecrosis of the femoral head. Eur J Clin Invest 2000;30(3): 215–21.
49. Mehsen N, Barnetche T, Redonnet-Vernhet I, et al. Coagulopathies frequency in aseptic osteonecrosis patients. Joint Bone Spine 2009;76(2):166–9.
50. Stowens DW, Teitelbaum SL, Kahn AJ, et al. Skeletal complications of Gaucher disease. Medicine 1985;64(5):310–22.

51. Sims KB, Pastores GM, Weinreb NJ, et al. Improvement of bone disease by imiglucerase (Cerezyme) therapy in patients with skeletal manifestations of type 1 Gaucher disease: results of a 48-month longitudinal cohort study. Clin Genet 2008;73(5):430–40.
52. Mont MA, Marulanda GA, Jones LC, et al. Systematic analysis of classification systems for osteonecrosis of the femoral head. J Bone Joint Surg Am 2006;88-A-(Suppl 3):16–26.
53. Glimcher MJ, Kenzora J. The biology of osteonecrosis of the human femoral head and its clinical implications: II. The pathological changes in the femoral head as an organ and in the hip joint. Clin Orthop Relat Res 1979;139:283–312.
54. Glimcher MJ, Kenzora J. The biology of osteonecrosis of the human femoral head and its clinical implications: I. Tissue biology. Clin Orthop Relat Res 1979;138:284–309.
55. Brown TD, Baker KJ, Brand RA. Structural consequences of subchondral bone involvement in segmental osteonecrosis of the femoral head. J Orthop Res 1992;10(1):79–97.
56. Takashima K, Sakai T, Hamada H, et al. Which classification system is most useful for classifying osteonecrosis of the femoral head? Clin Orthop Relat Res 2018;476(6):1240–9.
57. Oppermann J, Franzen J, Spies C, et al. The microvascular anatomy of the talus: a plastination study on the influence of total ankle replacement. Surg Radiol Anat 2014;36(5):487–94.
58. Gelberman R, Mortensen W. The arterial anatomy of the talus. Foot Ankle 1983;4(2):64–72.
59. Thordarson D, Triffon M, Terk M. Magnetic resonance imaging to detect avascular necrosis after open reduction and internal fixation of talar neck fractures. Foot Ankle Int 1996;17(12):742–7.
60. Babu N, Schuberth JM. Partial avascular necrosis after talar neck fracture. Foot Ankle Int 2010;31(9):777–80.
61. Sangeorzan B, Benirschke S, Mosca V, et al. Displaced intra-articular fractures of the tarsal navicular. J Bone Joint Surg Am 1989;71(10):1504–10.
62. Williams G, Cowell H. Köhlers disease of the tarsal navicular. Clin Orthop Relat Res 1981;158:53–8.
63. Mohiuddin T, Jennison T, Damany D. Muller-Weiss disease - review of current knowledge. Foot Ankle Surg 2014;20(2):79–84.
64. Maceira E, Rochera R. Müller-Weiss disease: clinical and biomechanical features. Foot Ankle Clin 2004;9(1):105–25.
65. Tan A, Smulders Y, Zöphel O. Use of remodeled femoral head allograft for tarsal reconstruction in the treatment of Müller-Weiss disease. J Foot Ankle Surg 2011;50:721–6.
66. Zimmer E. Diseases, injuries, and varieties of the tarsal navicular. Arch Orthop Trauma Surg 1937;38:396–411.
67. Waugh W. The ossification and vascularisation of the tarsal navicular and their relation to Kohler's disease. J Bone Joint Surg Br 1958;40-B:765–77.
68. Saxena A, Fullem B, Hannaford D. Results of treatment of 22 navicular stress fractures and a new proposed radiographic classification system. J Foot Ankle Surg 2000;39(2):96–103.
69. McKeon KE, McCormick JJ, Johnson JE, et al. Intraosseous and extraosseous arterial anatomy of the adult navicular. Foot Ankle Int 2012;33(10):857–61.
70. Fitch K, Blackwell J, Gilmour W. Operation for non-union of the tarsal navicular. J Bone Joint Surg Br 1989;71:105–10.

71. Kwon YU, Choi JS, Kong GM, et al. Idiopathic avascular necrosis of first meta-
    tarsal head in a pediatric patient. J Foot Ankle Surg 2017;56(3):683–6.
72. Suzuki J, Tanaka Y, Omokawa S, et al. Idiopathic osteonecrosis of the first meta-
    tarsal head: a case report. Clin Orthop Relat Res 2003;415:239–43.
73. Meier P, Kenzora J. The risks and benefits of distal first metatarsal osteotomy.
    Foot Ankle 1985;6:7–17.
74. Resch S, Stenström A, Gustafson T. Circulatory disturbance of the first metatarsal
    head after Chevron osteotomy as shown by bone scintigraphy. Foot Ankle 1992;
    13(3):137–42.
75. Shariff R, Attar F, Osarumwene D, et al. The risk of avascular necrosis following
    chevron osteotomy: a prospective study using bone scintigraphy. Acta Orthop
    Belg 2009;75(2):234–8.
76. Easley ME, Kelly IP. Avascular necrosis of the hallux metatarsal head. Foot Ankle
    Clin 2000;5(3):591–608.
77. Thomas R, Espinosa F, Richardson E. Radiographic changes in the first meta-
    tarsal head after distal chevron osteotomy combined with lateral release through
    a plantar approach. Foot Ankle Int 1994;15(6):285–92.
78. Shereff M, Yang Q, Kummer F. Extraosseous and intraosseous arterial supply to
    the first metatarsal and metatarsophalangeal joint. Foot Ankle 1987;8(2):81–93.
79. Malal JJ, Shaw-Dunn J, Kumar CS. Blood supply to the first metatarsal head and
    vessels at risk with a chevron osteotomy. J Bone Joint Surg Am 2007;89(9):
    2018–22.
80. Tonogai I, Wada K, Higashino K, et al. Location and direction of the nutrient artery
    to the first metatarsal at risk in osteotomy for hallux valgus. Foot Ankle Surg 2018;
    24(5):460–5 [Epub ahead of print].
81. Bayliss N, Klenerman L. Avascular necrosis of lesser metatarsal heads following
    forefoot surgery. Foot Ankle 1989;10(3):124–8.
82. Petersen WJ, Lankes JM, Paulsen F, et al. The arterial supply of the lesser meta-
    tarsal heads: a vascular injection study in human cadavers. Foot Ankle Int 2002;
    23(6):491–5.
83. Freiberg AH. Infraction of the second metatarsal bone, a typical injury. Surg Gy-
    necol Ostet 1914;19:191–3.
84. Gauthier G, Elbaz R. Freiberg's infraction: a subchondral bone fatigue fracture. A
    new surgical treatment. Clin Orthop Relat Res 1979;93:93–5.
85. Renander A. Two cases of typical osteochondropathy of the medial sesamoid
    bone of the first metatarsal. Acta Radiol 1924;3(6):521–7.
86. Waizy H, Jager M, Abbara-Czardybon M, et al. Surgical treatment of AVN of the
    fibular (lateral) sesamoid. Foot Ankle Int 2008;29(2):231–6.
87. Ogata K, Sugioka Y, Urano Y, et al. Idiopathic osteonecrosis of the first metatarsal
    sesamoid. Skeletal Radiol 1986;15:141–5.
88. Pretterklieber ML, Wanivenhaus A. The arterial supply of the sesamoid bones of
    the hallux: the course and source of the nutrient arteries as an anatomical basis
    for surgical approaches to the great toe. Foot Ankle 1992;13(1):27–31.
89. Rath B, Notermans HP, Frank D, et al. Arterial anatomy of the hallucal sesamoids.
    Clin Anat 2009;22(6):755–60.

Imaging Features of Avascular Necrosis of the Foot and Ankle

Spencer Couturier, MD, BS[a], Garry Gold, MD[b],*

KEYWORDS

- Avascular necrosis • Osteonecrosis • Talus • Müller-Weiss syndrome
- Freiberg infraction • MRI

KEY POINTS

- Avascular necrosis of the foot and ankle is a relatively rare entity that can affect any osseous structure in the foot or ankle but often manifests in typical locations.
- Recognition and understanding of key radiographic and early-stage MRI characteristics are essential to guide intervention.
- MRI is the most sensitive and specific imaging modality for characterizing early-stage avascular necrosis.
- Multimodality imaging features of avascular necrosis closely parallel the underlying pathophysiologic changes of avascular necrosis.

INTRODUCTION

Avascular necrosis (AVN) and osteonecrosis are both terms that imply bone death secondary to circulatory disturbance and are often used interchangeably in medical literature.[1] Historically osteonecrosis has been applied to describe ischemic bone death secondary to sepsis, whereas AVN denotes bone death that is both avascular and aseptic.[2] A wide variety of processes can result in disturbance of the vascular supply with subsequent deprivation of oxygen leading to AVN, including traumatic or compressive arterial inflow disruption, venous outflow obstruction, or intraluminal vascular occlusion. The femoral head, humeral head, scaphoid, and talus are the most common sites of AVN after traumatic disruption of the intramedullary blood supply.[1,3,4] AVN has been described in almost every bone of the ankle and foot, with

---

Dr G. Gold receives research support from GE Healthcare. Dr S. Couturier has nothing to disclose.

[a] Department of Radiology, Stanford University, Lane Building, 300 Pasteur Drive H0342, Stanford, CA 94305, USA; [b] Radiology and (by courtesy) Orthopedics and Bioengineering, Department of Radiology, Stanford University, 1201 Welch Road, Room P-263, Stanford, CA 94305, USA
* Corresponding author.
E-mail address: Gold@Stanford.edu

Foot Ankle Clin N Am 24 (2019) 17–33
https://doi.org/10.1016/j.fcl.2018.10.002

trauma the leading cause.[4] Nontraumatic causes of AVN include corticosteroids, alcoholism, hyperlipidemia, hemoglobinopathies, inherited thrombophilias, renal transplantation, diabetes, systemic lupus erythematosus (SLE), and irradiation.[2–4] A wide variety of systemic processes increase the risk of AVN, including sickle cell disease, SLE, diabetic ischemia, and corticosteroids. Multifocal infarctions of the foot and ankle are possible with systemic causes of AVN, although the talus and calcaneus are the most commonly affected sites.[5]

RADIOGRAPHIC AND COMPUTED TOMOGRAPHY IMAGING

AVN occurs when any portion of the vascular network is interrupted, including arteries, capillaries, sinusoids, and veins. Traditionally, the nature of the interruption can be classified as physical (trauma), compressive, or obstructive disruption of vessels.[6] All result in ischemic necrosis of the underlying bone when the vasculature can no longer supply sufficient oxygen.[7] In response to oxygen deprivation, the affected bones attempt repair via reossification, revascularization, and resorption of necrotic bone.[8] These processes result in predictable radiographic appearances of bones that are affected by AVN.

If imaged early, AVN can be radiographically occult. On early radiographic interrogation, the bones will often appear equal to adjacent bones in opacity. This lag time between the vascular insult and visible radiographic manifestations of AVN intimately mirrors the underlying pathophysiology. To cause AVN, an injury must disrupt vascular supply, resulting in hyperemia within perfused portions of the affected bone, leading to resorption of healthy bone. This resorption causes relative osteopenia. The osteopenia becomes more pronounced with further resorption, creating greater contrast between the remaining necrotic bone, which appears densely sclerotic (**Fig. 1**). Necrotic bone in the setting of AVN is unable to be resorbed due to inadequate vascular supply. Conspicuity of the necrotic bone will continue to increase as reossification takes place and new bone is laid down over necrotic trabeculae. The result is the typical sclerotic appearance of AVN (**Fig. 2**) on radiographs. In addition to changes of reossification, revascularization and resorption also tend to occur surrounding necrotic bone, which can result in a lucent rim around the area of osteonecrosis.[6–8]

The appearance of AVN on computed tomography (CT) mirrors that of radiography. Early CT imaging will often not demonstrate changes of AVN for the same reasons discussed previously. Resorption of healthy bone results in decreased Hounsfield units, reflecting osteopenia. During reossification, new bone is laid down over necrotic trabeculae, increasing Hounsfield units and sclerosis.

MRI

MRI is the most sensitive imaging modality for detection of early stage AVN. In addition to suggesting the diagnosis of AVN, MRI offers essential information to the orthopedic surgeon. Features, including the site and size of the involved segment, the presence of associated fractures, and the integrity of overlying articular cartilage and subchondral bone, affect clinical management.[5] These factors affect subsequent management decisions, including whether to perform core decompression, bone grafting, arthrodesis, or joint replacement.[5] The ankle is imaged in axial, coronal, and sagittal planes that are relative to the table top, whereas the foot is imaged in the oblique axial plane (parallel to the long axis of the metatarsal bones) and oblique sagittal plane. Elimination of magic angle artifact and optimal views of the peroneal tendons and the calcaneofibular ligament is achieved by placing the foot in approximately 20° of plantar flexion.[9] Intravenous gadolinium administration can aid in the assessment of the extent of

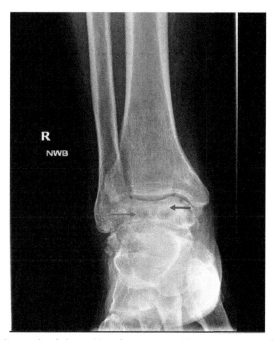

Fig. 1. Frontal radiograph of the ankle of a 45-year-old patient status after bone marrow transplant complicated by AVN of the talus. The radiograph demonstrates prominent central lucency within the talus (*blue arrow*), which represents healthy bone resorption. The adjacent sclerotic bone (*red arrow*) corresponds to necrotic bone that cannot be resorbed due to the lack of adequate blood supply.

nonenhancing infarcted bone, which may assist surgical planning; however, typically, gadolinium is not necessary when imaging AVN unless there is a high index of suspicion for hardware complication secondary to infection. Because many cases of AVN stem from traumatic injury, ferromagnetic screws and hardware are often within the field of view and can result in artifacts. The use of fast spin echo and short tau inversion recovery (STIR) sequences reduces metal-related artifacts compared with gradient echo and frequency-selective fat-saturation sequences.[3,10] An increase in susceptibility and misregistration artifacts has been observed with greater field strength (1.5 T to 3.0 T), although broader bandwidth and higher gradient field strengths can be used to offset the effect partially. At higher field strength, additional imaging parameter optimization steps include using a smaller field of view, increasing the resolution (matrix size), thinner slices, increasing the echo train length, and increasing the bandwidth. With more metal in place, multispectral MRI methods may be helpful in reducing artifacts.[11]

The earliest detectable evidence of AVN on MRI is bone marrow edema, which manifests as an ill-defined low signal on T1-weighted images with corresponding high signal on T2-weighted fluid-sensitive sequences (**Fig. 3**). Histologically, bone marrow edema correlates with ischemic death of hematopoietic cells, capillary endothelial cells, and lipocytes with a subsequent increase in extracellular fluid within the bone. Edema secondary to AVN will typically be present by the second week after the inciting vascular interruption.[3] In traumatic or early postoperative settings, marrow edema and hemorrhage also occur secondary to disruption of trabeculae and leakage

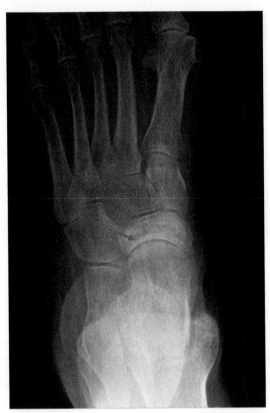

Fig. 2. Radiograph of the right foot of a 60-year-old patient who fell while ambulating 1 month before presentation demonstrates intense sclerosis (*blue arrow*) of the navicular bone without underlying fracture. Sclerosis corresponds with necrotic bone that cannot be resorbed due to vascular supply disruption.

of fluid and blood products into the extracellular space.[12] Thus, marrow edema-like signal is a nonspecific MRI finding that can be due to many causes; for example, hematopoietic marrow reconversion, infection, trauma, and malignancy.[13] Differentiating early AVN marrow edema signal from other causes is difficult. For example, after lower limb injury marrow edema patterns within the osseous structures of the foot and ankle are common, and often resolve after immobilization. According to Pearce and colleagues[2], subchondral and subcortical marrow edema often stabilized by 18 weeks, with no associated new pain or underlying clinical syndrome. Due to the lack of specificity, early bone marrow edema alone should be interpreted with caution, especially in the setting of trauma.

As changes of AVN occur and radiographically apparent sclerosis develops within the infarcted bone, low-signal intensity becomes visible on both T1-weighted and T2-weighted images. The interface between necrotic bone and viable granulation tissue manifests as the classically described double-line sign, a low-signal intensity rim within which the inner aspect demonstrates high signal on T2-weighted images (**Fig. 4**). Although characteristic of AVN within other sites of the body such as the humeral head and femur, the double-line sign is infrequently observed within the foot and ankle.

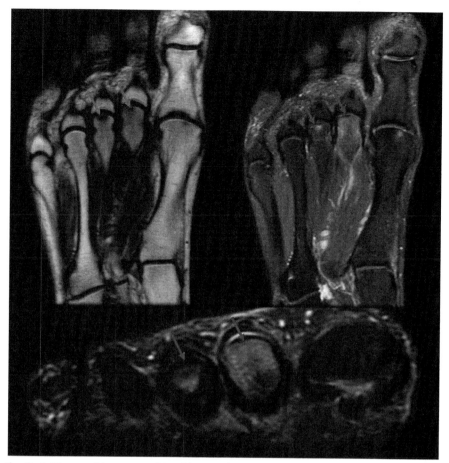

Fig. 3. A 55-year-old woman with a history of sarcoidosis on high-dose steroids who presented with chronic midfoot pain. T1-weighted images demonstrate focal low signal in the second and, to a lesser extent, the third metatarsal heads (*blue arrows, top right image*). T2-weighted images demonstrate corresponding high-signal (*red arrows, top left and bottom images*). No visible fracture line is evident. Imaging findings and clinical history are highly suggestive of AVN of the metatarsal heads.

TALAR AVASCULAR NECROSIS

Derived from the Latin word taxillus, talus originally referred to the ankle bone of a horse, which commonly served as playing dice for Roman soldiers.[1] The talus is the second largest of the tarsal bones and has a unique structure designed to channel and distribute body weight. Articular cartilage covers approximately 60% of its surface, and there are no muscular or tendinous attachments.[3,4] Consequently, only a limited area of penetrable bone is available for vascular perforation. This feature, combined with small nutrient vessels, variations in intraosseous anastomoses, and a lack of collateral circulation, predispose the talus to AVN when its vascular supply is disturbed. Furthermore, deposition of fibroadipose granulation tissue adjacent to necrotic bone and persistent mechanical stress may impair the ingrowth of new vessels, thereby preventing healing. Broadly, AVN of the talus fits into 3 categories:

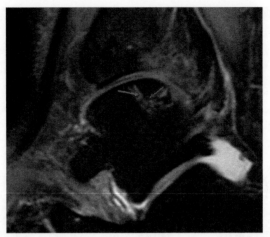

Fig. 4. T2-weighted image demonstrates changes of AVN involving the talar dome. The inner high-signal line (*blue arrow*) represents granulation tissue, and the internal low-signal line represents sclerotic bone (*red arrow*). This finding is known as the double-line sign.

traumatic, idiopathic, and medication-induced. Although a precise percentage is not well known, up to 75% of cases stem from traumatic causes. Of the remaining cases that are nontraumatic, AVN commonly results from renal or bone marrow transplantation (**Fig. 5**), as well as chronic steroid use (**Fig. 6**).[14]

In posttraumatic cases involving fractures of the distal tibia and talar neck, quantifying the effect of the initial traumatic disruption of blood supply as opposed to subsequent orthopedic intervention is difficult (**Figs. 7** and **8**). A further complicating

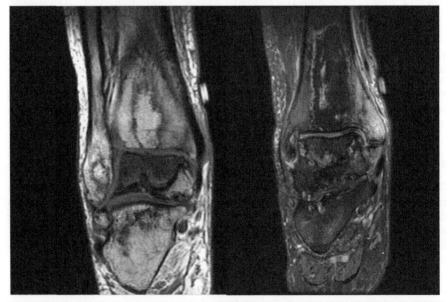

Fig. 5. 45-year-old patient status after bone marrow transplant. T1-weighted (*right*) and T2-proton-density-weighted (*left*) coronal images of the ankle demonstrate extensive changes of AVN in the talus, in addition to multifocal bone infarcts.

factor in assessing the pathogenesis and clinical prevalence of posttraumatic AVN is the observation that, although most cases of posttraumatic AVN of the foot manifest clinically within the first months after injury, cases in the distal tibial metaphysis may remain clinically asymptomatic.[4,15] Leland Hawkins[15] first described 3 critical patterns of talar neck injury, with a fourth pattern later added by Canale and Kelly.[2] This pattern-based system correlates the risk of vascular disruption and the risk of subsequent AVN with the degree of displacement and dislocation. Hawkins type 1 injuries are non-displaced talar neck fractures with 10% to 15% prevalence of AVN. Hawkins type 2 injuries represent displaced fractures combined with dislocation or subluxation of the subtalar joint with a 20% to 50% risk of AVN. Hawkins type 3 injuries are displaced fractures combined with dislocation or subluxation of both the ankle joint and subtalar joints, with the associated risk of AVN near 100% (**Fig. 9**). Type 4 injuries are displaced fractures with dislocation or subluxation of the subtalar, tibiotalar, and talonavicular joints, with a reported 100% risk of AVN.[2]

Radiographically, AVN of the talus often manifests as an area of increased sclerosis in the talar dome, which can also extend into the talar body. Collapse of the subarticular surface and, in severe cases, fragmentation of the talar dome and body also occurs (**Fig. 10**). Knowledge of the Hawkins classification system helps risk-stratify patients based on the radiographic extent of a traumatic injury before AVN develops. Although an in-depth review of talar anatomy is beyond the scope of this article, a few key definitions are paramount to the discussion. Talar anatomy is extensively studied, and ossification of the talus originates from a single primary center that induces elongation in an anteroposterior direction.[16] The talar frame, consisting of the body, neck, and head, articulates with the calcaneus inferiorly, the tibia and fibula superolaterally (proximally), and the navicular bone distally.[17,18] The body of the talus is uniquely shaped, being wider anteriorly than posteriorly. The posterior process comprises 2 tubercles that are divided by the groove of the flexor hallucis longus tendon. In approximately 50% of the general population, an os trigonum is present over the lateral tubercle.[19] The superolateral and, to a lesser extent, the medial cartilaginous surface

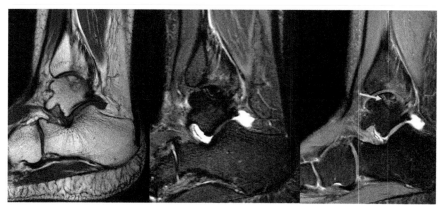

Fig. 6. A 26-year-old woman status after heart transplant complicated by rejection, on a chronic steroid treatment regimen with chronic ankle pain. The sagittal T1-weighted image demonstrates peripheral low-signal along the lateral talar dome (*blue arrow*) without associated subchondral fracture or articular collapse. Sagittal STIR (*red arrow*) and proton-density-weighted images (*yellow arrow*) demonstrate a corresponding high signal. Imaging findings and clinical history were compatible with medication (steroid)-induced AVN of the talus.

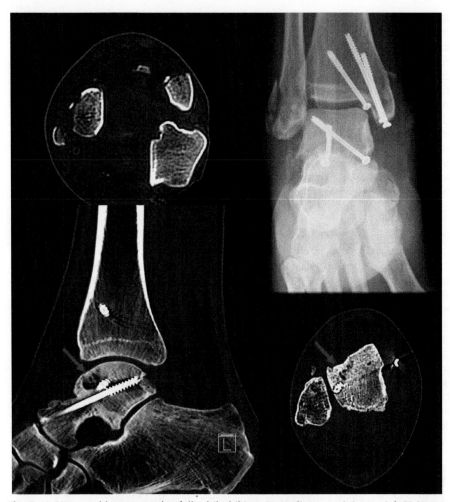

Fig. 7. A 27-year-old woman who fell while hiking. Immediate postinjury axial CT image (*top right*) demonstrates comminuted fracture deformities of the medial and lateral malleolus, disruption of the ankle mortise, with fracture and displacement of the talus. The corresponding postoperative radiograph (*top left*) demonstrates surgical reduction. Follow-up sagittal CT (*bottom right*) and axial CT images (*bottom left*) demonstrates focal lucency and adjacent sclerosis involving the lateral aspect of the talar articular surface, with 1 mm subarticular collapse (*red arrows*). Imaging features were compatible with a diagnosis of posttraumatic AVN of the talus.

of the talus extends to articulate with the tibia and fibula, whereas the inferior surface articulates with the posterior facet of the calcaneus, forming a portion of the subtalar joint.[16,20] The neck of the talus is narrowed superiorly, inferiorly, and laterally. Also, the talar neck has both a paucity of cartilage and a roughened appearance due to its many ligamentous insertions. The head of the talus is a convex structure with numerous articulations. Its anterior cartilaginous surface articulates with the navicular bone, whereas its inferomedial surface articulates with the anterior and middle facets of the calcaneus, the spring ligament, and the deltoid ligament.[16]

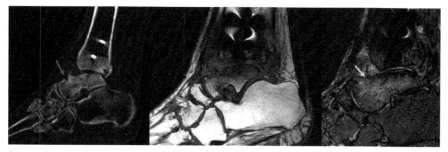

Fig. 8. A 60-year-old woman who slipped and suffered a bimalleolar fracture that was treated surgically, who presented with ongoing pain, and was diagnosed with AVN of the talus. Sagittal CT image demonstrates extensive subchondral sclerosis and fracture involving the talar dome (*blue arrow*) with multiple joint bodies. Sagittal T1-weighted image demonstrates low-signal (*red arrow*), and sagittal STIR image demonstrates high-signal corresponding with extensive reactive marrow edema (*yellow arrow*) and marked capsular thickening and synovitis involving the tibiotalar joint.

A talar neck fracture is present when the lateral fracture line starts in an extraarticular location at the lateral entrance to the tarsal sinus, regardless of extension into the anteromedial talar dome.[2] The position of the inferior fracture line is the most important feature that determines if the fracture extends into the talar body. If the fracture

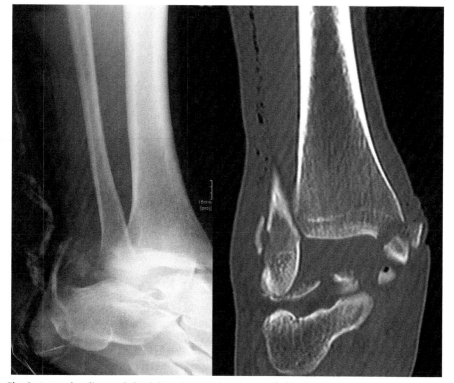

Fig. 9. Lateral radiograph (*right*) and coronal CT image (*left*) of the ankle demonstrate dislocation of both the ankle and subtalar joints in addition to extensive fracture deformities. Findings are compatible with a Hawkins type III injury, which carries a near 100% risk of developing AVN, which the patient subsequently developed (see **Fig. 7**).

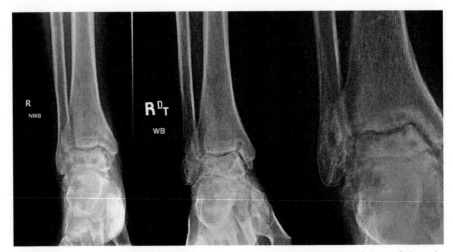

Fig. 10. Sequential radiographs of the ankle demonstrate progression of AVN of the talus (*progressing from right to left*). After 2-years, progressive irregularity and collapse of the talar dome is evident (*left*).

line involves the posterior facet of the talus, a fracture of the talar body is present. This subtle distinction carries significant prognostic weight because talar body fractures have a higher prevalence of AVN.[2]

Early AVN of the talus manifests as low signal on T1-weighted images, with high signal on T2-weighted images, in a typical marrow edema pattern. As viable granulation tissue and necrotic bone accumulate, a double-line sign appearance is possible (see previous discussion; see **Fig. 4**). When osteochondral fragmentation occurs, a rim sign can often be seen. A distinct finding, a rim sign appearance should not be confused with the double-line sign, because a rim sign implies instability. The rim sign comprises a high-signal T2-weighted line or an intermediate-signal T1-weighted line interposed between 2 low-signal lines. The central high-signal represents fluid between sclerotic borders of an osteochondral fragment (**Fig. 11**).

MÜLLER-WEISS SYNDROME

The navicular bone of the midfoot is the last bone in the foot to ossify. Classically described as boat-shaped, the navicular bone has multiple articulations with other structures in the midfoot. Proximally, it articulates with the head of the talus. Laterally, the navicular bone articulates with the cuboid bone. Distally, it articulates with the lateral, intermediate, and medial cuneiform bones. The dorsal cuneonavicular ligament and plantar cuneonavicular ligament connect each cuneiform to the navicular bone. The main vascular supply of the navicular bone is the dorsalis pedis artery.[21] Smaller branches of the medial plantar artery also supply the plantar aspects of the navicular bone.[22] Traumatic navicular bone fractures are relatively rare events but are more common than AVN.

Müller-Weiss syndrome is a rare condition of AVN that affects the tarsal navicular bone in adults and, although often used interchangeably with the term spontaneous osteonecrosis of the navicular bone, there is controversy concerning the cause of the disease. For example, pathologic evidence of AVN is not present in all specimens.[22,23] Müller-Weiss syndrome is a distinct and separate process from Köhler

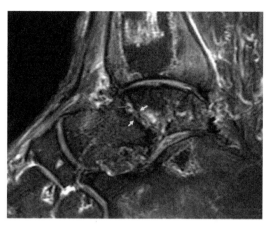

Fig. 11. Sagittal T2-weighted fat-saturation image of the ankle demonstrates extensive changes of AVN involving all of the visualized osseous structures. There is flattening and collapse of the talus (*blue arrow*). Fragmentation of the talus is also depicted with a rim sign appearance of central high-signal (*red arrow*) representing fluid insinuation between the sclerotic borders of osteochondral fragments, which are visualized as low-signal lines (*yellow arrows*).

disease, which typically affects children and is often a self-limited condition. Most often, Müller-Weiss presents with bilateral chronic dorsomedial midfoot pain without a clinically significant history of trauma.[24] Most commonly affecting women in the fifth decade of life, patients experience wide variance in clinical symptoms, ranging from asymptomatic to debilitating chronic pain. Weightbearing radiographs may demonstrate the diagnosis. Early stage radiographic images typically demonstrate decreased volume and increased sclerosis of the sclerosis of the lateral aspect of the navicular bone. As the condition progresses, the navicular bone assumes a comma shape morphology secondary to collapse of the lateral aspects (**Fig. 12**). Although not always seen, fragmentation of the navicular bone can occur. In the early stages, bone marrow edema in the lateral navicular bone may be visible as low-intensity T1-weighted signal and corresponding high-intensity T2-weighted signal. With the progression of AVN, the classic comma shape can also be observed on MRI with fragmentation and collapse of the lateral aspects of the navicular bone. As with talar AVN, low signal can develop on both T1-weighted and T2-weighted images as radiographically apparent sclerosis develops (**Figs. 13** and **14**). Conservative management with nonsteroidal antiinflammatory drugs or immobilization is often unsuccessful, often prompting surgical intervention. Left unchecked, chronic Müller-Weiss can progress to advanced midfoot osteoarthritis, resulting in permanent disability.[24,25]

FREIBERG INFRACTION

The 5 long bones of the foot numbered from one to 5; the metatarsals are comparable to the metacarpals of the hand. Each metatarsal has a base, a shaft, a neck, and a head which articulates with the articular surface of the adjacent phalange. Anatomically the first through third metatarsals contribute to the medial longitudinal arch, whereas the fourth and fifth metatarsals contribute to the lateral longitudinal arch. The bases of the 5 metatarsals form the transverse arch via articulation with the cuboid and cuneiform bones. Classically involving the second metatarsal head, Freiberg infarction results in subchondral collapse and changes of AVN (**Fig. 15**). Despite the

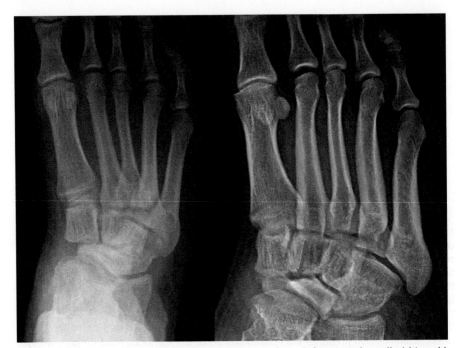

Fig. 12. A 36-year-old man with a history of chronic foot deformity who rolled his ankle while playing basketball. Initial radiograph (*right*) was obtained 8 weeks after initial injury and demonstrates sclerosis of the navicular bone with irregularity of the lateral aspect. Follow-up radiograph (*left*) 4 years postinjury demonstrate collapse of the lateral aspect of the navicular bone with intense sclerosis and a classic comma shape (*blue arrow*).

traditional association with the second metatarsal head, AVN can occur in any of the metatarsal heads. Although the definitive cause of Freiberg infraction is unknown, most suspect that it is a multifactorial process that may result from acute or repetitive stress trauma. Adolescent women are the most commonly affected demographic and, in some cases, high-heeled shoes can be a causative factor.[26] There is much overlap with metatarsal stress fracture with regard to both clinical symptomatology and imaging findings, especially early in the disease process.[27] As with other sites of AVN, early imaging findings include low-signal intensity within the affected metatarsal head on T1-weighted images with high-signal intensity on T2-weighted and STIR images (see **Fig. 3**).[28] As the infarction progresses, low-signal develops on T2-weighted images and collapse of the metatarsal head occurs. The low-signal on T2-weighted images corresponds with sclerosis on radiographs.[29]

SESAMOID AVASCULAR NECROSIS

The hallux sesamoids are the most common site of sesamoid AVN in the foot. Paired, ovoid ossicles of the great toe, the hallux sesamoids begin ossification in adolescence, usually around the eighth year of life. Most commonly, 2 distinct sesamoids are formed and embedded into the short flexor tendons of the great toe.[30] This anatomic positioning allows the sesamoids to act as a fulcrum, which increases the leverage of the flexor hallucis longus and brevis. The dorsal surface of the sesamoids articulates with the undersurface of the first metatarsal head, which has a grooved configuration. Arterial supply is often variant but the most common branches extend

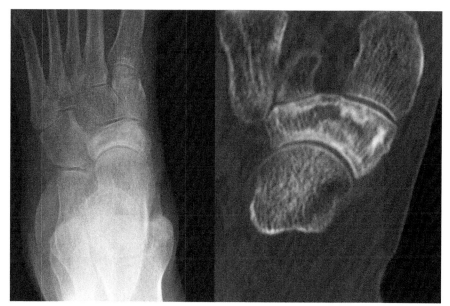

Fig. 13. Radiograph (*right*) and coronal CT image (*left*) of the right foot of a 60-year-old patient who fell while ambulating 1 month before presentation. Note the dense sclerotic changes in the navicular bone without a visible fracture or fragmentation (for corresponding MRI, see **Fig. 11**).

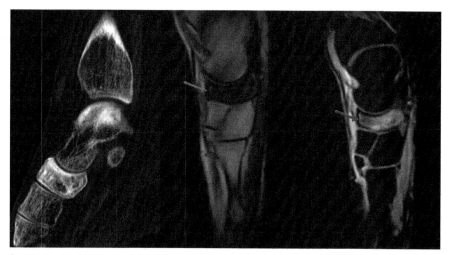

Fig. 14. Sagittal CT image (*right*) from the patient in **Fig. 9**, demonstrates profound sclerotic changes of the navicular bone. The T1-weighted sagittal image (*middle*) demonstrates low signal throughout the navicular bone (*blue arrow*) corresponding to radiographic sclerosis. A STIR sagittal image (*left*) also demonstrates a linear low signal corresponding to radiographic sclerosis (*red arrow*). Additional high signal is present, compatible with marrow edema. The patient was diagnosed with AVN of the navicular bone.

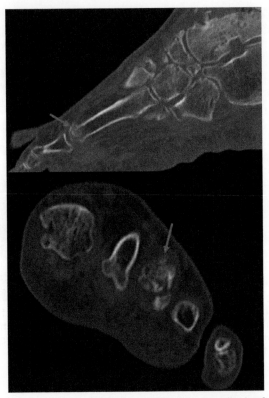

Fig. 15. A 60-year-old woman who slipped and suffered a bimalleolar fracture, which was treated with open reduction and internal fixation, who presented with ongoing pain. Sagittal (*top*) and Coronal (*bottom*) CT images demonstrate patchy sclerosis and lucency in the third metatarsal head, with flattening and cortical irregularity (*blue arrows*). The constellation of findings is suggestive of late-stage AVN of the third metatarsal head. Of note, the patient also has late-stage AVN of the talar dome (see **Fig. 8**).

from the medial plantar artery. Additional branches of the lateral plantar artery and the dorsalis pedis artery are also common. AVN of the sesamoid is relatively rare although likely underreported clinically. Patients often present with pain on direct palpation, aggravated by forced dorsiflexion of the great toe. Specific precipitating events include repetitive microtrauma from track and field, dance, and chronic foot alignment disorders.[31] If clinically suspected, weightbearing radiographs in multiple projections are of high clinical utility to evaluate for typical radiographic features of sesamoid AVN. Distinguishing multipartite sesamoids from fragmented sesamoids is critical. Multipartite hallux sesamoids are a common anatomic variant, present in up to 33% of normal sesamoids.[30] The tibial sided sesamoid is more commonly divided (bipartite) compared with the fibular-sided sesamoid. One proposed explanation for the increased incidence in the tibial sesamoid is the frequent presence of multiple ossification centers. Another proposed mechanism may relate to larger biomechanical forces exerted on the fibular sesamoid.[31] Bipartite hallux sesamoids are typically bilateral (70% of cases).[31] Two features that favor a bipartite hallux sesamoid as opposed to fragmentation are the transverse orientation of lucency, as well as smooth and well-corticated edges (**Fig. 16**). Typical radiographic features include fragmentation into 2

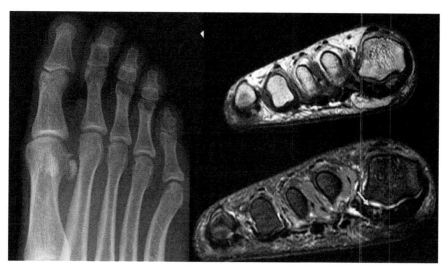

Fig. 16. A 21-year-old collegiate basketball player with pain overlying the first and second metatarsals for 2 weeks before presentation. Radiograph (*right*) demonstrates a multipartite fibular hallux sesamoid with irregular margins (*blue arrow*). The T1-weighted coronal image (*top left*) demonstrates diffuse low signal in the fibular hallux sesamoid (*red arrow*), with the corresponding high signal on the T2 weighted coronal image (*bottom left*) (*yellow arrow*). Imaging features are highly suggestive of AVN of the fibular hallux sesamoid.

or more pieces (with irregular edges), and the characteristic radiographic findings of AVN (see previous discussion), including relative osteopenia and increased sclerosis. MRI will often demonstrate the bone marrow edema pattern of low signal on T1-weighted images and corresponding high signal on STIR and T2-weighted images. As with other sites of AVN, low T2-signal will develop in regions of radiographically sclerosis (see **Fig. 13**).[31]

ACKNOWLEDGMENTS

The authors thank Kathryn Stevens, MD, for her contributions in the figures presented in this article.

REFERENCES

1. McCarthy I. The physiology of bone blood flow: a review. J Bone Joint Surg Am 2006;88:4–9.
2. Pearce DH, Mongiardi CN, Fornasier VL, et al. Avascular necrosis of the talus: a pictorial essay. Radiographics 2005;25(2):399–410.
3. Assouline-Dayan Y, Chang C, Greenspan A, et al. Pathogenesis and natural history of osteonecrosis. Semin Arthritis Rheum 2002;32(2):94–124.
4. DiGiovanni CW, Patel A, Calfee R, et al. Osteonecrosis in the foot. J Am Acad Orthop Surg 2007;15(4):208–17.
5. Koulouris G, Morrison WB. Foot and ankle disorders: radiographic signs. Semin Roentgenol 2005;40(4):358–79.
6. Resnick D, Sweet DE, Madewell JE. Osteonecrosis: pathogenesis, diagnostic techniques, specific situations, and complications. In: Diagnosis of bone and joint disorders. 4th edition. Philadelphia: Saunders; 2002. p. 3599–685.

7. Solomon L. Mechanisms of idiopathic osteonecrosis. Orthop Clin North Am 1985; 16:655–67. Medline.

8. Christman RA, Cohen R. Osteonecrosis and osteochondrosis. In: Foot and ankle radiology. St Louis (MO): Churchill Livingstone; 2003. p. 452–81.

9. Rosenberg ZS, Beltran J, Bencardino JT. From the RSNA refresher courses. Radiological Society of North America. MR imaging of the ankle and foot. Radiographics 2000;20:S153–79.

10. Steffen RT, Athanasou NA, Gill HS, et al. Avascular necrosis associated with fracture of femoral head after hip resurfacing. J Bone Joint Surg Br 2010;92(6): 787–93.

11. Koch KM, Bhave S, Gaddipati A, et al. Multispectral diffusion-weighted imaging near metal implants. Magn Reson Med 2017;79:987–93.

12. Bartoníček J, Fric V, Skála-Rosenbaum J, et al. Avascular necrosis of the femoral head in pertrochanteric fractures: a report of 8 cases and a review of the literature. J Orthop Trauma 2007;21(4):229–36.

13. Pape D, Seil R, Anagnostakos K, et al. Postarthroscopic osteonecrosis of the knee. Arthroscopy 2007;23(4):428–38.

14. Gross CE, Haughom B, Chahal J, et al. Treatments for avascular necrosis of the talus: a systematic review. Foot Ankle Spec 2014;7(5):387–97.

15. Hawkins L. Fractures of the neck of the talus. J Bone Joint Surg Am 1970;52(5): 991–1002.

16. Berquist TH. Radiology of the foot and ankle. 2nd edition. Philadelphia: Lippincott Williams & Wilkins; 2000. p. 218–24.

17. Bucholz RW, Heckman JD. Rockwood and Green's fractures in adults. Philadelphia: Lippincott Williams & Wilkins; 2001. p. 2091–129.

18. Canale ST, Kelly FB Jr. Fracture of the neck of the talus. J Bone Joint Surg Am 1978;60:143–56.

19. Lapidus PW. A note on the fracture of os trigonum: report of a case. Bull Hosp Joint Dis 1972;33:150–4.

20. Kleiger B, Ahmed M. Injuries of the talus and its joints. Clin Orthop 1976;121: 243–62.

21. Prathapamchandra V, Ravichandran P, Shanmugasundaram J, et al. Vascular foramina of navicular bone: a morphometric study. Anat Cell Biol 2017;50(2): 93–8.

22. Maceira E, Rochera R. Müller-Weiss disease: clinical and biomechanical features. Foot Ankle Clin 2004;9(1):105–25.

23. Nelson EW, Rivello GJ. Müller-Weiss disease of the tarsal navicular: an idiopathic case. J Foot Ankle Surg 2012;51(5):636–41.

24. Tosun B, Al F, Tosun A. Spontaneous osteonecrosis of the tarsal navicular in an adult: Mueller-Weiss syndrome. J Foot Ankle Surg 2011;50(2):221–4.

25. Kani KK, Mulcahy H, Chew FS. Case 228: Mueller-Weiss disease. Radiology 2016;279(1):317–21.

26. Katcherian DA. Treatment of Freiberg's disease. Orthop Clin North Am 1994;25: 69–81.

27. Chowchuen P, Resnick D. Stress fractures of the metatarsal heads. Skeletal Radiol 1998;27:22–5.

28. Resnick D, Kang HS. Internal derangement of joints: emphasis on MR imaging. Philadelphia: Saunders; 1997.

29. Ashman CJ, Klecker RJ, Yu JS. Forefoot pain involving the metatarsal region: differential diagnosis with MR imaging. Radiographics 2001;21(6):1425–40.

30. Taylor JA, Sartoris DJ, Huang GS, et al. Painful conditions affecting the first meta-tarsal sesamoid bones. Radiographics 1993;13(4):817–30.
31. Waizy H, Jager M, Abbara-Czardybon M, et al. Surgical treatment of AVN of the fibular (lateral) sesamoid. Foot Ankle Int 2008;29(2):231–6.

Natural History of Avascular Necrosis in the Talus

When to Operate

Andrew Haskell, MD

KEYWORDS

• Avascular necrosis • Osteonecrosis • AVN • Natural history • Talus

KEY POINTS

- The Ficat classification describes the current understanding of the natural history of avascular necrosis (AVN) of the talus, including preclinical, preradiographic, precollapse, post-collapse, and arthritic stages, though patients may remain at a stage for long periods of time.
- The natural history of patients with preradiographic or precollapse AVN likely depends on the size and location of the lesion.
- Symptoms do not correlate with stage, and patients may be minimally symptomatic despite diffuse involvement for long periods of time.
- Joint-sparing treatments hold promise to prevent collapse but none are universally successful.
- When structural collapse occurs, joint-sacrificing procedures may be needed to relieve symptoms.

INTRODUCTION

Avascular necrosis (AVN), or osteonecrosis, of the talus bone is a frequently progressive and often debilitating consequence of trauma, treatment with steroids, or a variety of other identified and unidentified risk factors. Patients may present for treatment before the structural integrity of the bone has been compromised, when joint-sparing strategies may facilitate restoration of normal bone, though none universally prevents progression of the disease.[1,2] When bone structure begins to fail, joint-sacrificing strategies, such as extensive hindfoot fusion or talar replacement, may be required to relieve symptoms.

Disclosure Statement: Dr A. Haskell is a consultant for Stryker, Inc and a shareholder for Ortho-Hub, Inc.
Departments of Orthopedic Surgery and Sports Medicine, Palo Alto Medical Foundation, 301 Industrial Road, San Carlos, CA 94070, USA
E-mail address: haskela@pamf.org

Foot Ankle Clin N Am 24 (2019) 35–45
https://doi.org/10.1016/j.fcl.2018.09.002
1083-7515/19/© 2018 Elsevier Inc. All rights reserved.

Understanding the natural history of a disease such as AVN may prevent unnecessary intervention in patients who would be expected to improve or, conversely, it may prevent a prolonged course of conservative care doomed to fail. Recognizing the consequence of inaction guides clinical decisions that are fundamentally based on the risks and benefits of intervention. For example, in the case of AVN of the talus, the decision to initiate invasive procedures in a patient with minimal symptoms and intact talar structure necessitates a clear understanding of the fate of the untreated portion of the talus.

Staging of a disease frequently mirrors progression of pathologic findings and often helps guide treatment decisions. In the case of talar AVN, staging may be radiographic, or based on tissue changes, and it may or may not correlate with symptoms. The most widely used, the Ficat classification, has been revised over the years as imaging modalities improved and a better understanding of AVN of the talus emerged. Its current incarnation includes stage 0 (preclinical), stage I (preradiographic), stage II (precollapse, with radiographic changes), transition phase (with flattening or crescent sign), stage III (collapse with intact surrounding joints), and stage IV (osteoarthritis).[3] Other classifications follow a similar pattern, outlining the progression of disease from earliest manifestations to end-stage collapse.[4]

Unfortunately, understanding of AVN of the talus remains incomplete. The true incidence and prevalence is unknown mainly because of the frequent late presentation of patients. Strategies for optimal treatment lack the benefit of high-level-of-evidence studies.[5] Case series, frequently with mixed treatment plans and limited by selection bias, form the bulk of information available to guide clinical decisions.

Despite these limitations, this article reviews the natural history of AVN of the talus with the goal of suggesting appropriate timing of various joint-preserving and joint-sacrificing interventions. Analyses are based on published studies and case series, and conclusions are often, by necessity, expert-opinion. Clinical decisions should continue to be tailored to each individual situation until higher quality treatment and outcome studies become available to inform a reliable treatment algorithm.

PATHOPHYSIOLOGY AND IMAGING

The primary pathophysiology of AVN is characterized by massive death of bone resulting in areas of necrosis. Although other processes, such as infection, osteoarthritis, fracture, osteochondritis dissecans, and tumor, may also contain regions of bone necrosis, these diseases should not be confused with AVN.[6] Microscopic findings progress from premature conversion to fatty bone marrow, bone resorption, and replacement with granular tissue; edema within the marrow; and, finally, sclerosis at the margins of live bone (repair interface).[7]

Radiographs of AVN are characterized by increased sclerosis or serpiginous regions of mixed lytic and sclerotic bone, frequently involving the femoral head but also seen in the metaphysis and epiphysis of the knee, ankle, shoulder, elbow, and wrist. As the disease progresses and structural integrity of the involved bone fails, subchondral collapse (crescent sign) followed by complete structural collapse and associated arthritic changes develop.[8]

The presence of subchondral osteopenia of the talar dome (Hawkins sign) on anteroposterior or mortise radiographs after trauma, typically seen 6 to 12 weeks after a talar neck fracture, should not be mistaken for AVN. It actually suggests restoration of bone viability owing to osteoclast-mediated disuse osteopenia[1,9] (**Fig. 1**). Hawkins sign has a sensitivity of 100% for detecting vascularity of the talus after trauma but

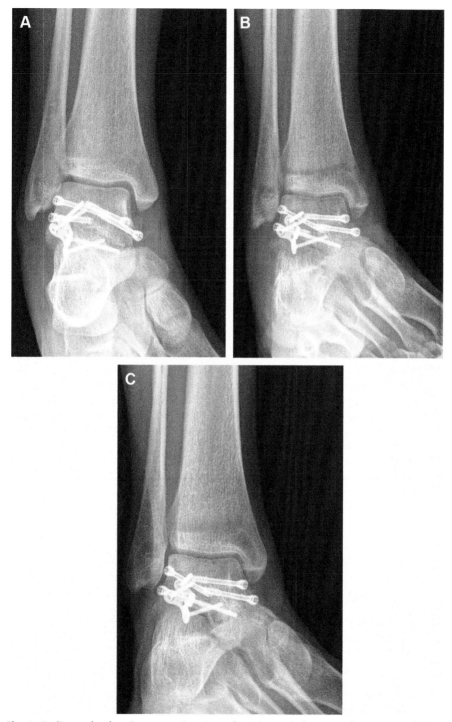

Fig. 1. Radiographs showing a mortise view of a talar neck fracture after open reduction and internal fixation at 1 week (*A*), 6 weeks (*B*), and 6 months (*C*). The periarticular osteopenia seen in the 6-week image (Hawkins sign) suggests adequate blood flow to the talus to allow osteoclast-mediated bone resorption related to disuse. By 6 months, the patient has been weightbearing and the periarticular osteopenia has resolved.

absence of Hawkins sign does not guarantee development of AVN because it has a specificity of only 58%.[9,10] Hawkins sign is present in 50%, 30%, and 33% of grade I, II, and III or IV talar neck fractures, whereas in the same cohort AVN developed in 0%, 10%, and 50% of these tali.[11]

MRI, computed tomography (CT), and bone scan supplement radiographs in the diagnosis of AVN. The degree and location of talar involvement may be characterized more completely with MRI than with standard radiographs.[12] MRI should be considered in high-risk patients with high clinical suspicion and negative radiographs, or posttraumatic patients with negative Hawkins sign. Hawkins stage I (preradiographic) AVN occurs because initial cell death may not be seen on MRI because lipid vacuoles in marrow adipocytes persist for a time even after cell death.[6] Preradiographic disease may be seen on MRI, with initial sclerotic changes seen at the margin of the lesion. This is followed by high signal at the inner border and low signal at the rim of the lesion; extension of increased T2 signal; and, finally, circumscribed regions of decreased T1 and T2 signals.[7] CT scan may also help identify the extent of AVN and show areas of early structural collapse.[8] Bone scintigraphy is used for early diagnosis, showing increased osteoblast activity and blood flow in early stages, and later decreased activity in the center of osteonecrotic regions. It can be used to assess disseminated AVN, though is less useful than CT or MRI at identifying extent of involvement in a single region of AVN.[13]

DEMOGRAPHICS AND ETIOLOGIC FACTORS

AVN of the talus is relatively rare, though the true prevalence is unknown. It accounts for a small percentage ($\sim$2%) of all symptomatic cases of AVN.[14] Patients with AVN of the talus are categorized into 2 distinct groups: those whose develop AVN after trauma and those without a history of trauma. A variety of risk factors have been identified for nontraumatic AVN, though none are exclusively causative, and presence of a risk factor is not a prerequisite for development. The final cause of AVN is an interruption to the blood supply to the bone, though the originating insult may be highly variable, depending on the patient's genetic predisposition, associated risk factors, and underlying medical conditions.[6,7]

Posttraumatic

Prior trauma is the leading cause of talar AVN, making up 75% of cases involving the talus.[15] Displaced fracture of the neck of the talus is the most common traumatic precursor, though other ankle and hindfoot trauma, and even minor injury, may also precede the diagnosis.[16] The age of patients with posttraumatic AVN varies widely, and men present more commonly than women.[9] It is typically unilateral, involving the injured ankle.

Risk of developing AVN of the talus is associated with the severity of the injury. The Hawkins classification of talar neck fractures describes increasing bone displacement and soft tissue injury with increasing grades.[1,9] As the grade increases, the risk of talar AVN rises: 0% to 13% in grade I injuries, 10% to 50% in grade II, and 50% to 91% in grade III.[1,9,11]

The increased risk of AVN of the talus with increasing displacement and soft tissue injury is likely related to the degree and duration of disruption to the blood supply to the talar body at the initial time of injury.[17] The timing of reduction or surgical fixation is not related to the risk of developing AVN.[18] Blood supply to the talus is limited by the high proportion of its surface that is articular, limiting entry for perforating vessels. The vasculature supplying the talus has been well-described. Most of the vasculature enters through the talar neck region through the tarsal sinus and the tarsal canal, which may explain the relationship between fractures of this region and AVN.[19–21]

However, injury severity does not entirely explain the natural history of the disease process in posttraumatic AVN of the talus. It is unclear why patients with seemingly similar degrees of bony displacement may have different outcomes. Perhaps the variability in vascular supply patterns to the talus spare some tali.[20,21] Possibly some intrinsic or extrinsic factors allow certain patients in the preradiographic stage to regain blood supply after an avascular episode.[22]

Nontraumatic

In some cases, AVN of the talus has no traumatic history and is typically associated with the systemic form, osteonecrosis. In these cases, a variety of medications, alcohol use, and systemic illnesses are known risk factors for development of AVN, responsible for about 25% of cases involving the talus.[15] The femoral head is the most commonly affected bone in nontraumatic AVN, and much of the understanding of AVN is based on study of this region. However, the systemic nature of the injury leads to multiple joint involvement in 63% of cases and bilateral involvement in 54% of cases.[14] Women present more commonly than men, and the age range of patients with nontraumatic AVN varies widely.[14]

The pathogenesis of nontraumatic AVN is incompletely understood, is likely multifactorial, and likely has numerous pathways leading to loss of blood supply to the bone. Vessels may be occluded by fat emboli, sickled red blood cells, or nitrogen bubbles (Caisson disease); they may clot in patients in a hypercoagulable state; or they may be externally compressed from elevated extraluminal pressure.[6] Systemic illnesses associated with AVN include systemic lupus erythematosus, sickle cell disease, scleroderma, diabetes, multiple sclerosis, and protein-S deficiency, though the association may be related to medications used to treat many of these illnesses.[14,23,24]

Oral corticosteroids are the medication most commonly associated with AVN. Both dosage and duration of steroid use affect the risk and severity of nontraumatic AVN.[14] The relationship of dosage and duration of steroid use and risk and severity of nontraumatic AVN could imply AVN is associated with a single episode of medication use, and the risk increases because the number of these single episodes increases. Alternatively, there could be an ongoing injury and repair cycle that is overwhelmed with increasing doses and duration. Patient factors surely predispose to higher or lower risk for developing AVN at similar dosing and duration.

Knowledge of patient factors predicting resilience or submission to injury is lacking. Patients typically develop nontraumatic AVN after steroid use within the first 6 months of beginning treatment, suggesting those at higher risk develop lesions early, and those at lower risk remain at low risk despite longer term use.[6] Lipid metabolism may also contribute to risk because statins have a protective effect in patients at risk for AVN from glucocorticoid use.[25] Patients with clinically relevant clotting disorders may decrease their risk of AVN progression with low-molecular-weight heparin. Perhaps subtle coagulopathies, hydration status, systemic hyperinflammatory state, or other factors explain why some patient would develop AVN, whereas other patients seem relatively immune to the disease.

NATURAL HISTORY AND TIMING OF TREATMENT

The Ficat classification provides an excellent overview of the current understanding of the natural history of AVN of the talus. When the disease is progressive, each stage inexorably leads to the next, from internal bone destruction to structural collapse and arthritis. However, the timing of this progression is variable, not all patients progress, and some may even recover.[3,6]

The type and magnitude of vascular disruption determines the natural course of disease. Knowing the exact moment of vascular insult allows insight into the natural history of posttraumatic AVN of the talus. Patients typically are followed radiographically after trauma, such as talar neck fracture, allowing diagnosis 6 weeks to 6 months after the initial trauma. In nontraumatic AVN, the timing from exposure to presentation is variable and patients may present in any stage of disease. Because the disease process begins close to the time of injury or exposure, if patients do not demonstrate avascular changes on imaging by 6 months, they are unlikely to develop AVN later.[6]

Lesion size also is likely determined around the time of initial injury or exposure. Lesions do not typically grow after or expand after the initial extent of damage becomes clear.[26] Some preradiographic lesions may even decrease in size or resolve, as shown in MRI studies of femoral head AVN.[22]

Recommendations for timing of intervention in AVN must be prefaced by an acknowledged lack of complete understanding of which patients may progress unrelentingly toward collapse and arthritis and which patients may experience a relatively long period of clinical and radiographic stability. Based on study of AVN of the hip, lack of pain may not be a good indicator of lack of progression risk. Joint-sparing procedures have been shown to minimize risk of progression and may be appropriate when balanced with the risk and morbidity of the specific intervention.[27]

If recovery is possible through intervention, the timing of intervention becomes critical because recovery of bony integrity never occurs after collapse commences. Joint-sparing procedures, particularly when associated with pain relief and especially when shown to reduce risk of disease progression, should be implemented before joint collapse is evident. The high complication rate of joint-sacrificing procedures accentuates the imperative to prevent collapse whenever possible.[5]

Stage 0 (Preclinical)

The natural history of preclinical nontraumatic AVN of the talus is difficult to characterize because patients typically only present for evaluation when they develop pain. Given that countless people are exposed to medication-associated or alcohol-associated risk factors each year, it is likely that some percentage of those exposed develop preclinical AVN and recover. What is uncertain is who is at risk of developing AVN, why some people resolve, and why others progress to become symptomatic. Genetic, environmental, nutritional, and local host factors all may play a role in determining who progresses to clinically relevant AVN.

Stage 1 (Preradiographic)

The natural history of patients with stage I (preradiographic) AVN is likely to depend on the size and location of the lesion. However, although characteristics of the lesion can influence the natural history, what determines these characteristics is unclear. Twenty-five subjects at risk for AVN with 32 asymptomatic hips demonstrating early changes on MRI were followed prospectively.[28] Smaller lesions away from the weightbearing, superior aspect of the head never progressed, whereas larger lesions involving the superior weightbearing aspect of the joint progressed to collapse (stage III) at an average of 15 months, with all collapsing by 4 years. In the talus, avascular change may be disseminated in the talar body or be focused, particularly to the anterior-lateral and superior aspect of the talar body, or even in the talar head.[29,30] Correlation of lesion size and location to risk of collapse in the talus is a logical extrapolation but has not been confirmed.

Stage 2 (Precollapse)

The natural history of patients with AVN of the talus who become symptomatic but have not collapsed (stage II) may best be characterized by persistence of symptoms and possible progression of disease when left untreated (**Fig. 2**). Twenty-nine ankles with Ficat stage 2 (precollapse) nontraumatic AVN of the talus, presenting an average of 5 months after symptoms began, were treated with 3 months of nonweightbearing; however, only 2 (7%) improved.[14]

Protecting tali with precollapse AVN from additional weightbearing-induced trauma for prolonged periods seems to improve clinical outcomes. Canale and Kelly[1] found that, after talar neck fractures, subjects with AVN treated with 9 or more months of nonweightbearing did better clinically than those treated with patellar tendon brace or shorter periods of protected weightbearing. Using Hawkins clinical grading scale, they reported 8 excellent, 4 good, 1 fair, and 0 poor results for prolonged (>9 months) nonweightbearing; 0 excellent, 2 good, 3 fair, and 1 poor results for patellar bracing; and 0 excellent, 2 good, 1 fair, and 5 poor results in subjects without restrictions. Hawkins[9] reported outcomes for subjects with posttraumatic talar AVN treated with nonweightbearing until fracture healing (presumably <9 months) of 1 excellent, 2 good, 12 fair, and 9 poor. Mindell and colleagues[31] reported collapse in 6 of 13 (46%) subjects with posttraumatic AVN of the talus allowed to bear weight at an average of 6 months and in all subjects before 9 months after injury. The lower risk of advancement to collapse in early-stage humeral head AVN further supports the association of weightbearing to progression.[32]

There is hope that joint-preserving treatments may alter the natural course of precollapse AVN of the talus, though high-level-of-evidence data are lacking. When considering using these modalities, intervene before progression to stage III (collapse) for best results. Alendronate, a bisphosphonate that improves bone density by diminishing the activity of osteoclasts, taken in combination with calcium and vitamin D3 for

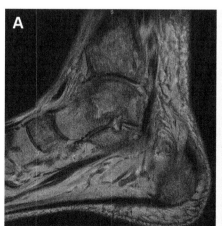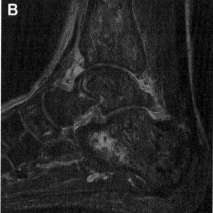

Fig. 2. Sagittal T1-weighted (*A*) and T2-weighted (*B*) MRI of an ankle with diffuse AVN involving multiple bones, including the tibia, talus, calcaneus, and navicular bones. The structure of the talus is intact and the joints are maintained, making this Ficat stage II (precollapse).

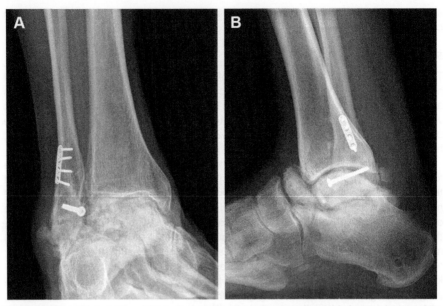

Fig. 3. Mortise (*A*) and lateral (*B*) radiographs of a posttraumatic case of AVN involving the talar body, associated with a nonunion of the talar neck and collapse of the talus. The joints are relatively nonarthritic, making this Ficat stage III (postcollapse).

3 years, improved symptoms and reduced femoral head collapse compared with historic controls at an average of 4 years.[33] Prospective randomized studies using pulsed electromagnetic field therapy in addition to other treatments found incremental improvement in pain relief and possible reduced risk of progression in early stage AVN of the hip.[34] Extracorporeal shockwave treatment has shown promise in AVN of the femoral head and talus.[5,35] Hyperbaric oxygen treatment in the early postoperative period has been described.[36] Injection with concentrated iliac crest bone marrow aspirate lowers the rate of collapse in precollapse posttraumatic AVN of the talus. Twelve of 45 (27%) subjects progressed to stage III after stem cell injection compared with 24 of 34 (71%) for controls treated with core decompression.[2]

More invasive joint-sparing procedures have also shown promise. Twenty-seven subjects with nontraumatic AVN of the talus treated with core drilling all avoided further operation at a mean of 7 years, though many remained symptomatic and 7 of 29 (24%) progressed to stage III (collapse).[14] In another series of 17 ankles undergoing core decompression, only 3 (18%) required fusion after an average of 7 years.[37] Vascularized bone graft transfer may help prevent collapse of early stage AVN of the talus.[38–41] Doi and Hattori[38] reported on 7 subjects who underwent transfer of vascularized bone from the supracondylar femur for precollapse talar body AVN with only 1 (14%) progressing to stage III (collapse).

Stage 3 and 4 (Postcollapse and Arthritis)

When patients develop structural collapse (Ficat stage III or IV), there is no chance of macrostructural restoration, though bony stability may be achieved, mitigating further collapse, and symptoms may be tolerable.[42] A period of nonweightbearing and joint-sparing procedures, such as core decompression, may provide symptomatic relief but are less successful than in stage II (precollapse) disease.[5,14]

If conservative treatments are unsuccessful, progression to definitive treatment with joint-sacrificing procedures frequently becomes necessary to resolve symptoms (**Fig. 3**). A variety of ankle and hindfoot fusion techniques have been described.[43–46] Consideration of ankle replacement or total talus replacement may be given in patients wishing to avoid fusion.[47–49] AVN of the talus with collapse is a contraindication for ankle replacement.

SUMMARY

AVN (osteonecrosis) of the talus may develop after a variety of traumatic and nontraumatic events interrupt the bone's vascular supply. The extent of involvement, and the risk and degree of progression from a structurally stable to a collapsed bone, is likely to be determined at the initial time of injury or exposure. Conservative measures, such as a period of nonweightbearing, in addition to surgical interventions, such as core drilling, bone grafting, and revascularization, may ultimately prove to alter the natural history of AVN. When collapse occurs, joint-sacrificing procedures, such as fusion, may be required to relieve symptoms. The relative rarity and variability of AVN makes comparative studies of treatments challenging.

REFERENCES

1. Canale ST, Kelly FB Jr. Fractures of the neck of the talus. Long-term evaluation of seventy-one cases. J Bone Joint Surg Am 1978;60(2):143–56.
2. Hernigou P, Dubory A, Flouzat Lachaniette CH, et al. Stem cell therapy in early post-traumatic talus osteonecrosis. Int Orthop 2018. https://doi.org/10.1007/s00264-017-3716-7.
3. Ficat RP. Idiopathic bone necrosis of the femoral head. Early diagnosis and treatment. J Bone Joint Surg Br 1985;67(1):3–9.
4. Steinberg ME, Steinberg DR. Classification systems for osteonecrosis: an overview. Orthop Clin North Am 2004;35(3):273–83, vii-viii.
5. Gross CE, Haughom B, Chahal J, et al. Treatments for avascular necrosis of the talus: a systematic review. Foot Ankle Spec 2014;7(5):387–97.
6. Lafforgue P. Pathophysiology and natural history of avascular necrosis of bone. Joint Bone Spine 2006;73(5):500–7.
7. Assouline-Dayan Y, Chang C, Greenspan A, et al. Pathogenesis and natural history of osteonecrosis. Semin Arthritis Rheum 2002;32(2):94–124.
8. Pearce DH, Mongiardi CN, Fornasier VL, et al. Avascular necrosis of the talus: a pictorial essay. Radiographics 2005;25(2):399–410.
9. Hawkins LG. Fractures of the neck of the talus. J Bone Joint Surg Am 1970;52(5):991–1002.
10. Tezval M, Dumont C, Sturmer KM. Prognostic reliability of the Hawkins sign in fractures of the talus. J Orthop Trauma 2007;21(8):538–43.
11. Chen H, Liu W, Deng L, et al. The prognostic value of the hawkins sign and diagnostic value of MRI after talar neck fractures. Foot Ankle Int 2014;35(12):1255–61.
12. Thordarson DB, Triffon MJ, Terk MR. Magnetic resonance imaging to detect avascular necrosis after open reduction and internal fixation of talar neck fractures. Foot Ankle Int 1996;17(12):742–7.
13. Bonnarens F, Hernandez A, D'Ambrosia R. Bone scintigraphic changes in osteonecrosis of the femoral head. Orthop Clin North Am 1985;16(4):697–703.
14. Delanois RE, Mont MA, Yoon TR, et al. Atraumatic osteonecrosis of the talus. J Bone Joint Surg Am 1998;80(4):529–36.

15. Adelaar RS, Madrian JR. Avascular necrosis of the talus. Orthop Clin North Am 2004;35(3):383–95, xi.
16. Feller JA, Hart JA, Doig SJ. Avascular necrosis of the talus following apparently minor ankle injury: a case report. Injury 1988;19(3):213–6.
17. Gillquist J, Oretop N, Stenstrom A, et al. Late results after vertical fracture of the talus. Injury 1974;6(2):173–9.
18. Buckwalter VJ, Westermann R, Mooers B, et al. Timing of surgical reduction and stabilization of talus fracture-dislocations. Am J Orthop (Belle Mead NJ) 2017; 46(6):E408–13.
19. Gelberman RH, Mortensen WW. The arterial anatomy of the talus. Foot Ankle 1983;4(2):64–72.
20. Miller AN, Prasarn ML, Dyke JP, et al. Quantitative assessment of the vascularity of the talus with gadolinium-enhanced magnetic resonance imaging. J Bone Joint Surg Am 2011;93(12):1116–21.
21. Prasarn ML, Miller AN, Dyke JP, et al. Arterial anatomy of the talus: a cadaver and gadolinium-enhanced MRI study. Foot Ankle Int 2010;31(11):987–93.
22. Kopecky KK, Braunstein EM, Brandt KD, et al. Apparent avascular necrosis of the hip: appearance and spontaneous resolution of MR findings in renal allograft recipients. Radiology 1991;179(2):523–7.
23. Tektonidou MG, Moutsopoulos HM. Immunologic factors in the pathogenesis of osteonecrosis. Orthop Clin North Am 2004;35(3):259–63, vii.
24. Korompilias AV, Ortel TL, Urbaniak JR. Coagulation abnormalities in patients with hip osteonecrosis. Orthop Clin North Am 2004;35(3):265–71, vii.
25. Pritchett JW. Statin therapy decreases the risk of osteonecrosis in patients receiving steroids. Clin Orthop Relat Res 2001;(386):173–8.
26. Shimizu K, Moriya H, Akita T, et al. Prediction of collapse with magnetic resonance imaging of avascular necrosis of the femoral head. J Bone Joint Surg Am 1994;76(2):215–23.
27. Belmar CJ, Steinberg ME, Hartman-Sloan KM. Does pain predict outcome in hips with osteonecrosis? Clin Orthop Relat Res 2004;425:158–62.
28. Takatori Y, Kokubo T, Ninomiya S, et al. Avascular necrosis of the femoral head. Natural history and magnetic resonance imaging. J Bone Joint Surg Br 1993; 75(2):217–21.
29. Babu N, Schuberth JM. Partial avascular necrosis after talar neck fracture. Foot Ankle Int 2010;31(9):777–80.
30. Schmidt DM, Romash MM. Atraumatic avascular necrosis of the head of the talus: a case report. Foot Ankle 1988;8(4):208–11.
31. Mindell ER, Cisek EE, Kartalian G, et al. Late results of injuries to the talus. analysis of forty cases. J Bone Joint Surg Am 1963;45(2):221–45.
32. Cruess RL. Steroid-induced avascular necrosis of the head of the humerus. Natural history and management. J Bone Joint Surg Br 1976;58(3):313–7.
33. Agarwala S, Shah S, Joshi VR. The use of alendronate in the treatment of avascular necrosis of the femoral head: follow-up to eight years. J Bone Joint Surg Br 2009;91(8):1013–8.
34. Al-Jabri T, Tan JYQ, Tong GY, et al. The role of electrical stimulation in the management of avascular necrosis of the femoral head in adults: a systematic review. BMC Musculoskelet Disord 2017;18(1):319.
35. Xie K, Mao Y, Qu X, et al. High-energy extracorporeal shock wave therapy for nontraumatic osteonecrosis of the femoral head. J Orthop Surg Res 2018; 13(1):25.

36. Mei-Dan O, Hetsroni I, Mann G, et al. Prevention of avascular necrosis in displaced talar neck fractures by hyperbaric oxygenation therapy: a dual case report. J Postgrad Med 2008;54(2):140–3.
37. Mont MA, Schon LC, Hungerford MW, et al. Avascular necrosis of the talus treated by core decompression. J Bone Joint Surg Br 1996;78(5):827–30.
38. Doi K, Hattori Y. Vascularized bone graft from the supracondylar region of the femur. Microsurgery 2009;29(5):379–84.
39. Rieger UM, Haug M, Schwarzl F, et al. Free microvascular iliac crest flap for extensive talar necrosis–case report with a 16-year long-term follow up. Microsurgery 2009;29(8):667–71.
40. Yu XG, Zhao DW, Sun Q, et al. [Treatment of non-traumatic avascular talar necrosis by transposition of vascularized cuneiform bone flap plus iliac cancellous bone grafting]. Zhonghua Yi Xue Za Zhi 2010;90(15):1035–8.
41. Kodama N, Takemura Y, Ueba H, et al. A new form of surgical treatment for patients with avascular necrosis of the talus and secondary osteoarthritis of the ankle. Bone Joint J 2015;97-B(6):802–8.
42. Churchill MA, Spencer JD. End-stage avascular necrosis of bone in renal transplant patients. The natural history. J Bone Joint Surg Br 1991;73(4):618–20.
43. Tenenbaum S, Stockton KG, Bariteau JT, et al. Salvage of avascular necrosis of the talus by combined ankle and hindfoot arthrodesis without structural bone graft. Foot Ankle Int 2015;36(3):282–7.
44. Dennison MG, Pool RD, Simonis RB, et al. Tibiocalcaneal fusion for avascular necrosis of the talus. J Bone Joint Surg Br 2001;83(2):199–203.
45. Devries JG, Philbin TM, Hyer CF. Retrograde intramedullary nail arthrodesis for avascular necrosis of the talus. Foot Ankle Int 2010;31(11):965–72.
46. Kendal AR, Cooke P, Sharp R. Arthroscopic ankle fusion for avascular necrosis of the talus. Foot Ankle Int 2015;36(5):591–7.
47. Harnroongroj T, Vanadurongwan V. The talar body prosthesis. J Bone Joint Surg Am 1997;79(9):1313–22.
48. Lee KB, Cho SG, Jung ST, et al. Total ankle arthroplasty following revascularization of avascular necrosis of the talar body: two case reports and literature review. Foot Ankle Int 2008;29(8):852–8.
49. de Sousa RJ, Rodrigues Pinto RP, de Oliveira Massada MM, et al. Hybrid ankle prosthesis in a case of post-traumatic avascular necrosis of the talus. Rev Bras Ortop 2011;46(1):94–6.

Prevention of Avascular Necrosis with Fractures of the Talar Neck

Michael P. Clare, MD[a],*, Patrick J. Maloney, MD[b]

KEYWORDS

- Talar neck fracture • Avascular necrosis of talus • Hawkins sign

KEY POINTS

- Displaced talar neck fractures are no longer a surgical emergency; timing of definitive surgery has no influence on development of avascular necrosis.
- Amount of initial fracture displacement is best predictor of osteonecrosis.
- Grossly displaced fractures or fracture-dislocations should be provisionally reduced, with or without temporary external fixation.
- Soft tissue stripping should be limited to whatever is necessary to obtain proper fracture reduction; dissection within the sinus tarsi and tarsal canal should be avoided.
- Rigid internal fixation with solid cortical screws, countersunk within talar head and placed "below the equator" to provide optimum mechanical stability.

INTRODUCTION

Fractures of the talar neck remain among the most challenging of injuries in the lower extremity. These fractures are typically the result of high-energy trauma, particularly motor vehicle collisions and falls from a height, in which a dorsally directed axial load applied to the plantar surface of the foot at the moment of impact forcibly traps the neck of the talus against the anterior margin of the tibial plafond. Talar neck injuries are functionally problematic, in that the talus represents the critical link among the ankle, subtalar, and talonavicular joints, such that these fractures often represent a 3-joint injury.

The inherent vascular supply to the talar body is particularly tenuous, as there are no muscle or tendon attachments to the talus, and approximately two-thirds of the surface area of the talus is covered by articular cartilage. The vascular supply derives

Disclosures: The authors have nothing to disclose.
[a] Foot & Ankle Fellowship, Florida Orthopaedic Institute, 13020 Telecom Parkway North, Tampa, FL 33637, USA; [b] The Institute for Foot and Ankle Reconstruction at Mercy, 301 St Paul Place, Baltimore, MD 21202, USA
* Corresponding author.
E-mail address: mpclaremd@gmail.com

primarily from an extraosseous anastamotic ring formed from branches of the posterior tibial, dorsalis pedis, and peroneal arteries, respectively.[1,2] Fractures of the talar neck presumably disrupt this anastamotic ring, and therefore much of the vascular supply to the talar body, which can pose significant potential problems in bone healing and overall integrity of the talus.

Osteonecrosis is among the most disastrous of complications following fractures of the talar neck, and can be functionally devastating to the involved limb. The extent of involvement within the talar body may vary from partial without collapse to complete with full collapse, depending on the severity of vascular damage. What follows is a description of injury factors, surgical factors, and postoperative factors that the orthopedic surgeon should thoroughly understand so as to minimize the risk of avascular necrosis with fractures of the talar neck.

INJURY FACTORS
Timing of Definitive Fixation

Displaced fractures of the talar neck have historically represented a true surgical emergency, in which surgical treatment was indicated within 6 to 8 hours of injury, wherever possible. Avascular necrosis rates with displaced fractures historically ranged from 70% to 100%, although fixation techniques used in these studies was primitive and typically consisted of Steinmann pins.[3,4]

More modern studies (using modern fixation) have since shown that the specific timing of definitive fixation (before or after 6–8 hours) has no particular bearing on the development of osteonecrosis.[5–7] In many instances, these patients were polytrauma patients with multiple injuries and were treated at high-volume trauma centers, such that definitive fixation was not always possible within the requisite time window.

Extent of Initial Displacement

It has long been shown that the most predictive factor associated with the development of avascular necrosis with fractures of the talar neck is the extent of initial displacement.[3–7] Intuitively, the greater the extent of initial fracture displacement, to the point of dislocation, the greater the extent of damage to the surrounding soft tissue envelope and concomitant disruption of the extraosseous vascular supply to the talar body. More recent studies[5–7] use dual-incision open reduction and modern internal fixation techniques, and found that osteonecrosis in displaced talar neck fractures occurred in up to 50% of cases, and was more frequent in those with greater initial displacement, including dislocation.

Vallier and colleagues,[8] in a separate large series of talar neck/body fractures, further subdivided the Hawkins type-II fractures into type-IIA (without subtalar dislocation) and type-IIB (with subtalar dislocation). They found that the presence of a concomitant subtalar dislocation was predictive of avascular necrosis. They reported a 0% incidence of osteonecrosis in type-IIA fractures, a 25% incidence in type-IIB fractures, and a 41% incidence in type-III patterns.

Provisional Reduction/Temporary External Fixation

Although the definitive treatment of displaced talar neck fractures is no longer a surgical emergency, and the timing of definitive surgery has no real impact on the development of osteonecrosis, the presence of significant fracture displacement with or without dislocation should still be addressed expeditiously. As with any grossly displaced fracture or dislocation, the increased local pressure from the involved fragment can lead to compromise of the surrounding soft tissue envelope and potential skin necrosis.

In the event of a displaced fracture or fracture-dislocation of the talar neck, immediate closed reduction should be attempted. The reduction maneuver consists of longitudinal traction with extreme plantarflexion, with manipulation of the midfoot (and therefore the talar head fragment) to align it with the hindfoot (talar body). With an associated subtalar dislocation, the heel should be manipulated into inversion or eversion, depending on the direction of the dislocation. Postreduction radiographs are obtained, and so long as the talus is "in the ballpark" (grossly aligned) with no residual underlying deformity or areas of potential soft tissue compromise, the limb can be immobilized in a splint and definitive surgery undertaken at a later date.

Closed reduction may not be possible with certain patterns, particularly the Hawkins type-III or type-IV patterns. In these instances, a percutaneous, mini-open, or formal open reduction may be necessary to provisionally align the fracture fragments. In these grossly unstable patterns, a temporizing delta-type external fixator frame can be invaluable to provisionally stabilize the limb and immobilize the surrounding soft tissue envelope (**Fig. 1**A–E). In this manner, computed tomography scanning or other advanced imaging studies can be obtained where needed, as part of preoperative planning. Definitive surgery can then be scheduled electively using the treating orthopedic surgeon's regular surgical team, as a means of optimizing surgical execution and maximizing overall patient outcome.

Alternatively, if the patient presents at a reasonable time of day, and both the treating surgeon and his or her regular surgical team is available, definitive treatment may be undertaken acutely.

SURGICAL FACTORS
Two-Incision Approach

Dual anteromedial and anterolateral incisions are the most commonly used surgical approach to the talar neck. The anteromedial incision extends from the tip of the medial malleolus in line with the medial column of the foot to a point just beyond the navicular tubercle (**Fig. 2**). In this manner, the deep dissection will course through the "soft spot" between the anterior and posterior tibial tendons, and posterior to the saphenous nerve and vein. The approach is potentially extensile, as it can be extended proximally to allow for a medial malleolar osteotomy for those patterns extending into the talar body or posteromedial process, as well as distally for access to the entire medial column of the foot as necessary (**Fig. 3**).

The anterolateral approach actually consists of the Böhler approach, coursing from the anterolateral corner of the ankle joint in line with the extensor digitorum longus and peroneus tertius tendons toward the base of the fourth metatarsal (**Fig. 4**). This approach is also considered extensile, as it can be extended proximally to allow for exposure of the lateral talar dome, with or without a lateral malleolar osteotomy, and distally for exposure of the entire lateral column of the foot as necessary.

ANTEROLATERAL (BÖHLER) APPROACH

We prefer completing the anterolateral approach first because most of the comminution is typically found medially, thus the most accurate initial indication of the extent of fracture displacement or rotational malalignment is found laterally. Hence, the anterolateral approach is initiated, and superficial dissection continues to the extensor retinaculum and tendon sheath of the extensor digitorum longus and peroneus tertius tendons. Care is taken to avoid violation of the superficial peroneal nerve proximally, although the proximal portion of the incision rarely extends proximal enough to visualize the nerve before it begins coursing medially toward the first ray.

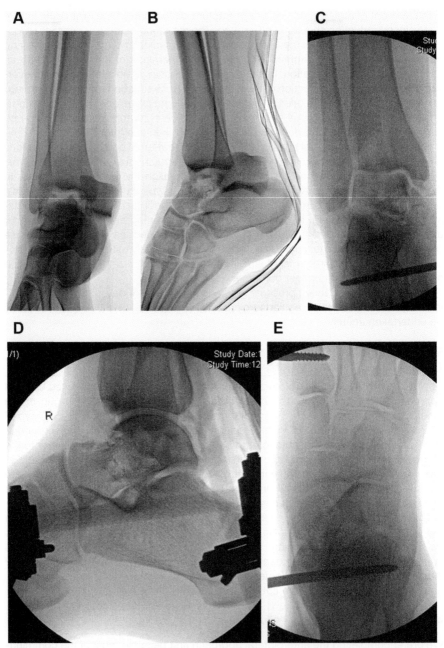

Fig. 1. (*A–E*) Hawkins 3 talar neck fracture-dislocation. (*A, B*) Ankle mortise and lateral injury radiographs. Note irreducible medial dislocation of talar body. (*C–E*) Intraoperative ankle mortise, lateral and anteroposterior foot views following formal open reduction and temporizing external fixation. Provisional alignment has been restored.

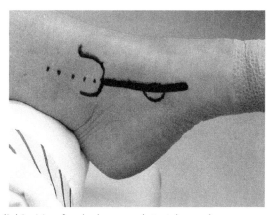

Fig. 2. Anteromedial incision for dual approach to talar neck.

The tendon sheath is incised at the lateral margin of the tendons and deep dissection is continued to the joint capsules of the ankle and subtalar joints proximally, and the extensor digitorum brevis muscle distally. The extensor brevis muscle is then traced to its origin beneath the tendons working dorsally, and subsequently reflected plantarly, thereby exposing the lateral capsule of the talonavicular joint and distal portion of the talar neck. The capsules of the ankle and subtalar joints are then released in line with and including the talonavicular joint capsule extending dorsally and plantarly, thereby completing a full-thickness flap (**Fig. 5**).

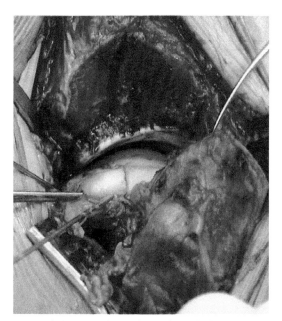

Fig. 3. Extensile anteromedial approach to talus with medial malleolar osteotomy. Note full visualization of talar body.

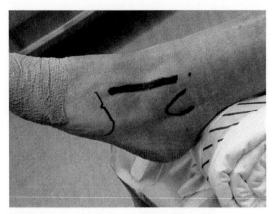

Fig. 4. Anterolateral incision for dual approach to talar neck.

Anteromedial Approach

The anteromedial approach is then initiated, and superficial dissection continues to the extensor retinaculum and joint capsule of the ankle joint proximally, and dorsal margin of the posterior tibial tendon sheath distally. The extensor retinaculum and capsules are longitudinally incised, continuing along the dorsal edge of the posterior tibial tendon through the underlying talonavicular joint capsule. Care is taken to avoid violation of the deltoid ligament fibers at the proximal margin of the incision.

The talonavicular joint capsule is then elevated in subperiosteal fashion off of the navicular tubercle, extending roughly to the midpoint of the navicular dorsally. The dorsal-most portion of the posterior tibial tendon insertion may also be reflected plantarly to ease soft tissue tension as necessary (**Fig. 6**). At the completion of the anterolateral and anteromedial approaches, the fracture pattern traversing the dorsal portion of talar neck should be easily visualized.

Limited Soft Tissue Stripping

As with the surgical management of most any fracture, limited soft tissue stripping is of paramount importance as a means of preserving periosteal blood supply to the

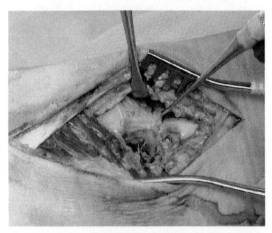

Fig. 5. Anterolateral approach to talus. Note exposure of talar head for eventual implant placement.

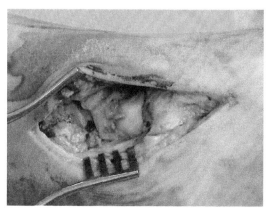

Fig. 6. Anteromedial approach to talus. Note exposure of talar head for eventual placement.

involved fracture fragments. Specific to the talar neck, every effort should be made to preserve the dorsal capsular reflection between the ankle and talonavicular joints, in an attempt to preserve as much inherent vascularity as possible. This capsular reflection represents an additional source of retrograde vascular supply to the talar body that should therefore be preserved wherever possible.

Limited Sinus Tarsi Dissection

In creating full-thickness flaps with the dual anterolateral and anteromedial approaches, there exists a delicate balance between completing sufficient dissection to expose the fracture fragments to facilitate fracture reduction, and performing excessive soft tissue stripping to where vascularity of the fragments and/or talar body is compromised.

We make a conscious effort to limit the extent of subperiosteal dissection into the sinus tarsi laterally and undersurface of the talar neck medially, exposing only what is necessary to obtain an anatomic reduction, so as to minimize further compromise of the already precarious blood supply to the talar body.

Rigid Internal Fixation

If the dual anteromedial and anterolateral approaches are properly performed extending through the talonavicular capsule medially and laterally, the foot may be adducted to expose the lateral portion of the talar head, and abducted to expose the medial portion of the talar head, which facilitates eventual screw placement.

Following reduction and provisional stabilization, solid cortical screws are placed in anterior to posterior fashion, countersunk within the talar head. In this manner, the trajectory of the implants will be as perpendicular to plane of the fracture line(s) as possible, thereby providing optimal stability. It is additionally imperative to place screws at or below the "equator" of the talar head, as plantar as possible within the talar head without violating the subtalar joint, to provide maximum stability on the tension side of the injury (**Fig. 7**). We prefer 3.5-mm to 4.0-mm cortical lag screws in the absence of comminution; in the event of comminution (typically medially), cortical position screws are used. Minifragment bridge plates can additionally be used in the event of severe comminution (**Fig. 8**).

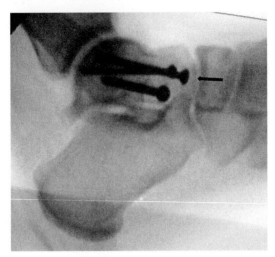

Fig. 7. Cortical screw fixation of a talar neck fracture countersunk within the talar head. Note that the screws are at or below the "equator" (*black arrow*) of the talar head for optimum stability.

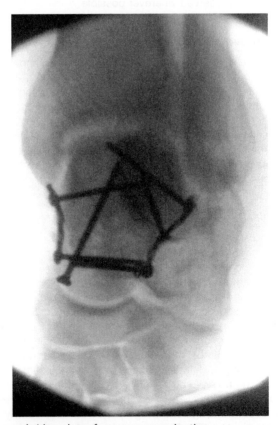

Fig. 8. Minifragment bridge plates for severe comminution.

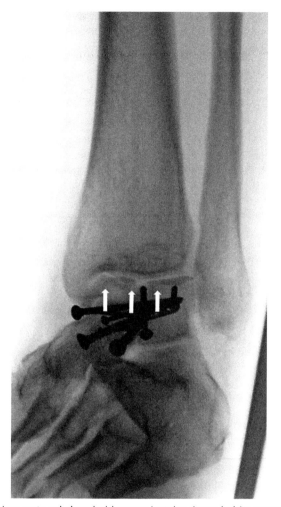

Fig. 9. Hawkins sign: note subchondral lucency in talar dome (*white arrows*).

POSTOPERATIVE FACTORS
Hawkins Sign

The Hawkins sign refers to subchondral lucency beneath the superior dome of the talus, best seen on a mortise view of the ankle (**Fig. 9**). The presence of a Hawkins sign is a favorable prognostic sign that osteonecrosis will not develop, but is not predictive of functional outcome.[9] The presence of a Hawkins sign has been shown to have a sensitivity of 100%, and specificity of 58%.[10] The timing of a Hawkins sign is typically 6 to 8 weeks postoperatively, but may require up to a year following surgery. The absence of a Hawkins sign long-term suggests that avascular necrosis has developed, although the talar body may not necessarily collapse.[8]

Postoperative Protocol/Time to Weightbearing

The involved limb is immobilized in a well-padded splint for the first 2 weeks to facilitate incisional healing, followed by conversion to a compression stocking and prefabricated fracture boot. Sutures are typically removed at 2 to 4 weeks following surgery. Range-of-motion exercises are initiated once the wounds are sealed and dry. Weight bearing is not generally permitted until 10 to 12 weeks following surgery, at which point there should be radiographic signs of healing. Progression of weight bearing does not require the presence of a Hawkins sign, as there is no clear correlation as to onset of weight bearing and the risk of osteonecrosis.[11]

SUMMARY

The timing of definitive surgery for displaced talar neck fractures has no bearing on the risk of osteonecrosis. The single best predictor of avascular necrosis is the amount of initial displacement. Grossly displaced fractures or fracture-dislocations should be provisionally reduced, with or without temporary external fixation. Periosteal stripping should be limited to only that which is necessary to obtain an anatomic reduction. Dissection within the sinus tarsi or tarsal canal should be avoided. Rigid internal fixation should be used, with solid cortical screws countersunk within the talar head and placed at or below the "equator" of the talar head for optimum stability. Bridge plating may be used for areas of comminution.

REFERENCES

1. Wildenauer E. Die Blutversorgung der Talus. Z Orthop Ihre Granzgeb 1975;113: 730.
2. Haliburton RA, Sullivan CR, Kelly PJ, et al. The extra-osseous and intra-osseous blood supply of the talus. J Bone Joint Surg Am 1958;40:1115–20.
3. Hawkins LG. Fractures of the neck of the talus. J Bone Joint Surg Am 1970;52: 991–1002.
4. Canale ST, Kelly FB Jr. Fractures of the neck of the talus: long term evaluation of seventy-one cases. J Bone Joint Surg Am 1978;60:143–56.
5. Lindvall E, Haidukewych G, Dipasquale T, et al. Open reduction and stable fixation of isolated, displaced talar neck and body fractures. J Bone Joint Surg Am 2004;86:2229–34.
6. Sanders DW, Busam M, Hattwick E, et al. Functional outcomes following displaced talar neck fractures. J Orthop Trauma 2004;18:265–70.
7. Vallier HA, Nork SE, Barei DP, et al. Talar neck fractures: results and outcomes. J Bone Joint Surg Am 2004;86:1616–24.
8. Vallier HA, Reichard SG, Boyd AJ, et al. A new look at the Hawkins classification for talar neck fractures: which features of injury and treatment are predictive of osteonecrosis? J Bone Joint Surg Am 2014;96:192–7.
9. Chen H, Liu W, Deng L, et al. The prognostic value of the Hawkins sign and diagnostic value of MRI after talar neck fractures. Foot Ankle Int 2014;35:1255–61.
10. Tezval M, Dumont C, Stürmer KM. Prognostic reliability of the Hawkins sign in fractures of the talus. J Orthop Trauma 2007;21:538–43.
11. Adelaar RS, Madrian JR. Avascular necrosis of the talus. Orthop Clin North Am 2004;35:383–95.

Avascular Necrosis of the Sesamoids

Kimberly Bartosiak, MD, Jeremy J. McCormick, MD*

KEYWORDS

- Sesamoid • Avascular • Osteonecrosis • Sesamoidectomy • Nonunion

KEY POINTS

- Avascular necrosis (AVN) of the sesamoid develops as a result of anatomic and mechanical factors as well as recurrent microtrauma.
- Sesamoid AVN is most commonly diagnosed with low signal intensity on T1 and T2 MRI studies along with late-stage radiographic fragmentation.
- Nonoperative treatment of sesamoid AVN is aimed at offloading the involved sesamoid with a protective boot or orthotic and has an unclear rate of success.
- Operative treatment of sesamoid AVN involves excision of the involved sesamoid and results most commonly in complete satisfaction and resolution of pain.
- Complications include hallux varus and hallux valgus as well as loss of push-off strength.

INTRODUCTION

Avascular necrosis (AVN) of the sesamoid bones of the great toe is a rare diagnosis. It was originally described in 1924 by Axel Renander. Initially referring only to the medial sesamoid, it was termed "Morbus Renander."[1] AVN of the sesamoids can be a difficult diagnosis to delineate with overlap of fracture, pseudoarthrosis, nonunion, and purely atraumatic AVN of the bone. The cause of sesamoid AVN could stem from any of the above mentioned or be secondary to isolated perfusion deficit or mechanical overload.[2] Repetitive microtrauma resulting in fracture or stress fracture with subsequent nonunion that evolves into avascular bone could also be considered a possible cause for this diagnosis. This article focuses on the evaluation, diagnosis, and treatment of medial and lateral sesamoid AVN.

DISCUSSION
Anatomy

The first metatarsophalangeal (MTP) joint is stabilized by a confluence of the collateral ligaments, plantar plate, abductor hallucis, adductor hallucis, and flexor hallucis brevis

The authors have nothing to disclose.
Department of Orthopaedic Surgery, Washington University School of Medicine, Campus Box 8233, 660 Euclid Avenue, St Louis, MO 63110, USA
* Corresponding author.
E-mail address: mccormickj@wustl.edu

Foot Ankle Clin N Am 24 (2019) 57–67
https://doi.org/10.1016/j.fcl.2018.09.004
1083-7515/19/© 2018 Elsevier Inc. All rights reserved.

(FHB). The FHB originates from the plantar aspect of the cuboid as well as medial, middle, and lateral cuneiforms. As it moves distally the FHB divides into medial and lateral slips that encompass each respective sesamoid. At the articulation of the sesamoids with the first metatarsal, the medial and lateral slips of FHB combine with the abductor and adductor hallucis tendons, respectively. Distal to the sesamoids the FHB tendons then combine with the plantar plate to insert on the base of the proximal phalanx as part of the capsular ligamentous complex (**Fig. 1**).[3]

The sesamoids ossify between ages 9 and 14 years with multipartite sesamoids present in 30% of individuals.[4] The medial sesamoid is the larger of the 2 and is positioned more directly under the metatarsal head resulting in increased weight-bearing forces on the medial compared with the lateral sesamoid.[5] This increased contact force is exacerbated by natural pronation of the first metatarsal and can be further increased in a cavus foot.[4] Despite these increased forces on the medial sesamoid, it is unclear which sesamoid has a higher prevalence of AVN, thus more than mechanical factors likely contribute to the development of this pathology. Contradicting studies exist, which do not agree on the predominant pattern of involvement, reporting medial, lateral, and even bilateral AVN as the most prevalent pattern depending on the reference.[5–10] Thus, it is unclear, given the low prevalence of sesamoid AVN, which sesamoid is at greater risk. Development of sesamoid AVN is likely multifactorial based on microtrauma, anatomic predispositions, and mechanical considerations including foot posture and activity profile.

Each sesamoid is supplied primarily by the first plantar metatarsal artery, a direct branch of the medial plantar artery off of the posterior tibial artery. There are also contributions from the plantar arch.[11] Vascularity of the sesamoids has been evaluated in

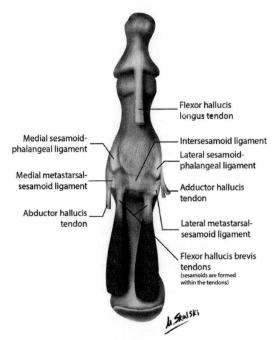

Fig. 1. Plantar view of the hallux MTP joint. (*From* Schein AJ, Skalski MR, Patel DB, et al. Turf toe and sesamoiditis: what the radiologist needs to know. Clin Imaging 2015;39:381; with permission.)

a series of cadaver studies with slightly differing conclusions. In a 1990 anatomic study of 13 subjects, Pretterklieber found a single vessel was responsible for perfusion of 63% of medial sesamoids with the lateral sesamoid supplied by a single vessel in 58% of feet.[12] Further anatomic studies of 29 feet by Pretterklieber and Wanivenhaus in 1992 demonstrated that in approximately half of feet branches from both the plantar arch and the medial plantar artery contributed equally to the vascular supply of the sesamoids. In approximately one-fourth of feet in the study, the major supply was from the medial plantar artery and in the remaining one-fourth of feet, from the plantar arch.[13] It has also been shown that the medial and lateral capsules contain sources of perfusion to each sesamoid.[14] Regardless of which artery is serving as the predominant source, the major supply enters antegrade at the plantar aspect of the bone, with the minor supply entering distally and supplying the sesamoids in a retrograde fashion through the distal capsular attachments.[11,15] Thus, the distal perfusion is more tenuous. Based on anatomic considerations alone the distal aspect of the sesamoid is more likely to develop AVN.

Pathologic evaluation of the abnormal sesamoid after surgical excision is not necessary. If, however, one were to section and examine the sesamoid under a microscope, the histology of AVN of the sesamoid displays characteristic AVN findings. This includes eosinophilic osteonecrosis with an absence of osteocytes. The bony trabecula will demonstrate necrosis and proliferation of granulation tissue (**Fig. 2**).[4]

PATIENT EVALUATION
History

AVN of a sesamoid occurs most commonly in women in the second or third decade of life. Patients may relate development of pain to increased activity or a particular minor trauma. The patient presents with symptoms of pain at the plantar aspect of the first metatarsophalangeal joint, with or without swelling.[5,16] Typical pain will be worse with weight bearing and with the last phase of the walking cycle. This may result in patients reporting walking on the lateral border of their foot in a pain avoidance gait pattern. Plantar pain often limits participation in activities or sports. All athletes are at risk but female ballet dancers have particularly high prevalence due to chronic microtrauma associated with sudden decelerations and foot positions resulting in high contact pressures on the sesamoids.[2,17] Patients have often modified their activities or

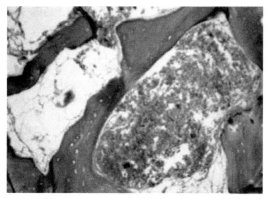

Fig. 2. Histologic section of hematoxylin-eosin–stained necrotic sesamoid. (*From* Toussirot E, Jeunet L, Michel F, et al. Avascular necrosis of the hallucal sesamoids update with reference to two case-reports. Joint Bone Spine 2003;70:308; with permission.)

shoe wear by the time of presentation with resultant improvement in symptoms with offloading. Unfortunately, the patient will often describe worsening symptoms on return to normal activities and baseline shoe wear.

Physical

On examination of the involved foot, inspection may identify a lateral callosity on the foot that develops secondary to a pain-avoidant gait pattern. Vascular examination would typically exhibit a palpable dorsalis pedis and posterior tibial artery as long as there is no concomitant vascular pathology. On sensory examination, one would not expect any deficit. It is important to assess the medial plantar nerve distribution, as surgical incisions could potentially lead to disruption in this distribution. On motor examination, one should assess the patient's ability to contract the extensor and flexor to the great toe and identify any pain associated with this motion. Remaining motor examination about the foot and ankle would be expected to be normal and painless.

When palpating the foot, the patient will endorse focal tenderness to palpation at the plantar aspect of the first MTP. It is critical to isolate the sesamoid on clinical examination that is symptomatic. There may be focused swelling in this area and the patient will experience increased pain with dorsiflexion and plantarflexion of the great toe. The pain is typically worse with passive dorsiflexion of the great toe.[4] Pain with range of motion may cause a limitation in both active and passive range of motion but without a firm endpoint as in hallux rigidus.

Posture and stability of the great toe should be assessed, paying close attention to any subtle hallux valgus or varus alignment, which will be important to note before any surgical intervention. The posture of the foot itself is more commonly cavus because this increases stress on the sesamoids as discussed previously. An assessment of gastrocnemius or Achilles tightness should be performed because the presence of equinus can contribute to increased pressures on the sesamoids during gait activities. When observing gait, patients may avoid loading the sesamoids by rolling to the outer border of the foot, which may result in transfer metatarsalgia. On completion of the history and physical examination, the differential diagnosis should be narrowed to include sesamoiditis, stress fracture, painful nonunion, osteomyelitis, symptomatic bipartite, and sesamoid AVN.

Radiographs

Initial radiographic views for a patient with pain over the sesamoids should include standard weight-bearing anteroposterior, oblique, and lateral foot radiographs as well as an axial sesamoid or Walter-Muller view. Plain radiographic findings are often delayed as with AVN in other anatomic areas. Once AVN has become a more longstanding issue for the patient, the axial sesamoid view will typically display a fragmented sesamoid with areas of demineralization or heterogenous striped sclerosis **(Fig. 3)**.[18] MRI can be obtained in these patients to help clarify or confirm the diagnosis, especially if the radiograph does not show clear pathology. MRI signal abnormalities develop within days of osteonecrosis occurring, making MRI particularly useful before development of radiographic changes or in the setting of a fragmented sesamoid to delineate between bipartite, nonunion, and AVN. In cases of AVN, the MRI will display low signal intensity on T1 and T2 as fibrous tissue replaces fat and hematopoietic tissue **(Fig. 4)**.[4] Normal bone marrow signal on T1-weighted sequences can exclude the diagnosis of osteonecrosis.[19] Fat subtraction or short tau inversion recovery (STIR) findings may demonstrate rim enhancement.[4] The diagnosis can be achieved without use of contrast.[19] Radiographs and MRI are most commonly used to help determine diagnosis for pain about the sesamoids.

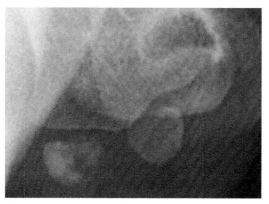

Fig. 3. Axial sesamoid view demonstrating lateral sesamoid fragmentation and sclerosis.

Computed tomography (CT) can be considered as an additional imaging modality.[18] This test adds little information to diagnosis but does help identify the number and character of fragments that can be helpful if planning sesamoidectomy to ensure all unhealthy fragments are identified and excised. Three-phase bone scintigraphy is less commonly used due to the high sensitivity of MRI scans but can be helpful in elucidating different diagnoses about the sesamoids. This is particularly helpful in situations when previous imaging has not demonstrated pathology or symptoms have not been present for an extended duration of time. Given the potential for delay in diagnosis by the above imaging modalities, bone scintigraphy can help provide an earlier diagnosis. Findings on bone scintigraphy characteristic of early AVN can include either low uptake or high uptake focused in the involved sesamoid without involvement of the MTP joint.[20]

Nonoperative Management

If a patient with focal sesamoid pain has not attempted nonoperative treatment before clinic presentation, this should trialed before considering operative intervention.

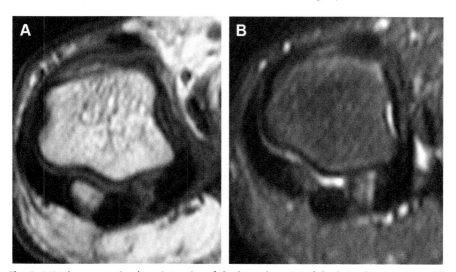

Fig. 4. MRI demonstrating hypointensity of the lateral aspect of the lateral sesamoid on (A) T1- and (B) T2-weighted imaging.

Swelling and pain can be addressed with basic rest, ice, compression, and elevation as well as nonsteroidal antiinflammatory medications.[3] A walking boot or walking short leg cast can be considered initially, particularly if the patient has significant swelling or acute onset of pain. The patient should be instructed on appropriate shoe wear, avoiding heeled shoes that would increase load on the forefoot. The shoe modifications can include orthotics that have an excavation under the metatarsal head to provide sesamoid relief, but patients may also consider an off-the-shelf turf toe plate or a custom Morton extension. These both will allow for limitation of hallux MTP dorsiflexion. If a more rigid construct is successful in alleviating symptoms then a patient can consider a custom shoe modification to stiffen the sole of the shoe.

Some advocate for non–weight-bearing for up to 6 months but given the typical presentation of these young active patients, prolonged non–weight-bearing can result in considerable deconditioning and may not be acceptable.[3,4,21] Steroid or lidocaine injections are not recommended, but if a patient is looking to maximize nonoperative interventions, particularly at the end of a season, a single judicious injection could be considered. Given the low prevalence of sesamoid AVN the success rate of nonoperative modalities is unknown. The decision to advance to surgical intervention should be made collectively between the patient and the physician after nonoperative management has failed to return the patient to an acceptable level of function and after an informed discussion of the risks and benefits of surgery.

Operative Management

Once nonoperative management has failed and a collective decision by the patient and provider has been made to pursue operative treatment, there is one mainstay of surgical treatment: sesamoidectomy of the involved sesamoid.

Lateral (fibular) sesamoid

Excision of the lateral sesamoid can be accomplished by either a dorsal or a plantar approach. It can be difficult to perform a lateral sesamoidectomy through a dorsal approach with a small intermetatarsal (IM 1–2) angle. If this angle is sufficient the lateral sesamoid can be laterally subluxated and accessed dorsally through the first web space. To accomplish this, a dorsal incision is made in the first web space. Using a lamina spreader, the first and second metatarsal heads are spread, the adductor hallucis is visualized, released, and subsequently the sesamoid can be shelled out of the FHB tendon.

The authors advocate for the more commonly used plantar approach. This approach significantly decreases lateral soft tissue disruption, allows visualization and protection of the plantar-lateral digital nerve (**Fig. 5**), and allows for repair of FHB. To excise the lateral sesamoid through a plantar approach, a curvilinear incision is made lateral to the weight-bearing pad of the hallux MTP joint. The sesamoid is excised by carefully shelling it from the FHB tendon using a beaver blade. The FHB tendon is then carefully repaired. The FHL must be identified and carefully protected. One must also be careful with this approach to have meticulous wound closure to reduce the risk of hypertrophic scar on the plantar weight-bearing aspect of the foot.[3]

Medial (tibial) sesamoid

Excision of the medial sesamoid can be accomplished through a plantar-medial approach. A medial incision is centered just proximal to the hallux MTP. The plantar-medial digital nerve (**Fig. 6**) is identified and protected and subsequently the medial sesamoid is identified. If an intraarticular approach is necessary to access all diseased fragments from intraarticular view, the capsule is incised along the superior

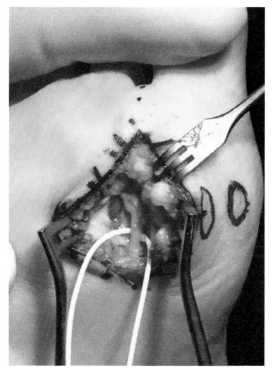

Fig. 5. Lateral sesamoidectomy plantar view with vessel loop around the plantar lateral digital nerve.

border of the abductor hallucis. The authors prefer an extraarticular approach with a careful longitudinal incision and reflection of periosteum on the plantar aspect of the sesamoid (**Fig. 7**). This allows for the FHB to be repaired after sesamoidectomy. The FHL must be carefully protected throughout this procedure as well.[3]

Rarely would excision of both sesamoids be indicated. In the instance of medial and lateral sesamoid pathology the recommendation would be to do a staged procedure. Excise the more symptomatic sesamoid and then, after an appropriate recovery period, determine if symptoms have resolved before considering removing the remaining sesamoid. This is an extremely rare circumstance, most commonly a result

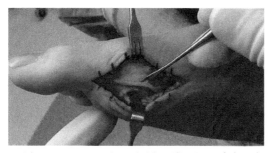

Fig. 6. Medial sesamoidectomy approach with identification of the plantar-medial digital nerve.

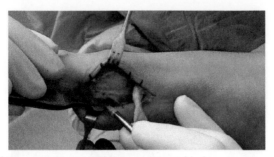

Fig. 7. Excision of the medial sesamoid using a Beaver blade.

of hallux dislocation. Sesamoidectomy of both medial and lateral sesamoids can result in a cock-up deformity. To prevent this complication, it is critical to repair the FHB and consider abductor transfer to the more plantar aspect of the hallux MTP joint in the void left by the medial sesamoid (**Fig. 8**).[3] Interphalangeal joint fusion has also been used if both sesamoids are excised to prevent clawing.[22]

After a sesamoidectomy, a patient will often develop loss of push-off strength. This is typically not noticeable in a nonathlete, but if the patient is a dancer or athlete reliant on push-off strength at the first MTP, this deficit may be obvious.[3] Strength is more affected with lateral sesamoidectomy with 16% loss of push-off strength compared with 10% with medial sesamoidectomy. With both sesamoids excised, 30% of push-off strength is compromised.[23] The other major concern with sesamoidectomy is hallux valgus and varus with medial and lateral sesamoidectomy, respectively. If a hallux valgus deformity exists at time of sesamoidectomy it should be addressed simultaneously. Careful soft tissue management and repair intraoperatively as well as a careful postoperative dressing and care is critical to preventing development of hallux varus or valgus. Finally, after medial sesamoidectomy, a defect in plantar soft tissues can be augmented by transferring the abductor hallucis tendon into the defect after releasing its distal insertion as mentioned earlier.[3]

Postoperative Management

After sesamoidectomy, the first MTP is carefully dressed and splinted in slight plantar flexion. The first MTP is also held in a slight varus position following medial sesamoidectomy to avoid stretching the repair and prevent development of hallux valgus. Alternatively, following lateral sesamoidectomy, the first MTP is held in slight valgus

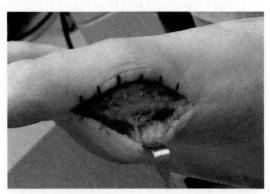

Fig. 8. Abductor repair into defect following medial sesamoidectomy.

position to prevent development of hallux varus. Given the plantar-based incision typically used for lateral sesamoidectomy, the patient is kept non–weight-bearing or heel-touch weight-bearing for 2 weeks or until the wound has healed. If the wound has healed and sutures are removed, weight-bearing may begin at 2 weeks in a walking boot with transition to a hard-soled shoe at 6 weeks. Sutures are often left in for an extended period of 3 to 4 weeks to assure appropriate skin apposition and healing. Following medial sesamoidectomy the patient may be protected weight-bearing in a walking boot or postoperative shoe. Following suture removal at approximately 2 weeks, the patient can be weight-bearing to tolerance in a walking boot with a removable bunion splint until 6 weeks after surgery.[3]

Following removal of the initial postoperative splint or dressing after medial or lateral sesamoidectomy, gentle passive range of motion may begin. Early motion will decrease risk of developing arthrofibrosis at the sesamoid-first MTP articulation. Therapy and active range of motion may be started when sutures are removed. Typically, a patient will begin to wean from their boot or postop shoe around 6 weeks after surgery. At that point they may begin a progressive rehabilitation protocol, starting with low-impact exercise in the form or bicycle or elliptical, and moving to a light jog and run if low-impact activities are well tolerated. Patients may be able to return to sport at around 3 months after surgery. The authors suggest athletes use a turf toe plate and/or protective taping with their shoe wear when returning to activity.[3]

Outcomes

Results following sesamoidectomy were initially published in 1933 by Inge and Ferguson in a study of 41 feet on 31 patients. This study demonstrated 42% of patients with complete relief and 29% with some relief. In their patient cohort only one lateral sesamoidectomy was performed, 15 feet underwent medial sesamoidectomy, and the remaining 25 feet had both sesamoids excised. Three of the five patients who reported no improvement had both medial and lateral sesamoids excised simultaneously.[24]

Mann published similar results in 1985 in a series of 21 sesamoidectomies. In this series 19 of 21 patients demonstrated some improvement with only 50% experiencing complete relief. Range of motion was compromised postoperatively in 34% of patients. When tested postoperatively, 12 of these patients demonstrated push-off or great toe flexion weakness, but this was not always clinically noticeable. Hallux valgus developed in 1 of 13 patients following medial sesamoidectomy. One of eight patients who underwent lateral sesamoidectomy developed hallux varus.[25] Leventen in 1991 demonstrated more promising results with complete satisfaction demonstrated in 18 of 23 patients and suggested sesamoidectomy as a safe and simple procedure with a predictable satisfactory outcome.[6]

SUMMARY

AVN of the sesamoid involves mechanical and anatomic predisposition combined with recurrent microtrauma. Most often the clinical diagnosis is made by history and physical examination, where a patient describes plantar first MTP joint pain and examination demonstrates focal pain over the involved sesamoid. Radiographs can show fragmentation and striped sclerosis. MRI findings are consistent with AVN in other anatomic areas. Bone scintigraphy and CT are used rarely. Treatment options include offloading the first MTP with an orthotic or walking boot and, if conservative measures fail, excising the involved sesamoid. Patients undergoing sesamoidectomy for AVN are most commonly satisfied with their outcomes following surgery.

REFERENCES

1. Renander A. Two cases of typical osteochondropathy of the medial sesamoid bone of the first metatarsal. Acta Radiol 1924;3:521–7.
2. Kalweit M, Frank D. Die aseptische Nekrose des Sesambeines am Metatarsale I – (Morbus Renander) –: Ein FallberichtAseptic necrosis of the first metatarsal sesamoid (Morbus Renander). FussSprungg 2003;1:148–51.
3. McCormick JJ, Anderson RB. The great toe: failed turf toe, chronic turf toe, and complicated sesamoid injuries. Foot Ankle Clin 2009;14(2):135–50.
4. Toussirot E, Jeunet L, Michel F, et al. Avascular necrosis of the hallucal sesamoids update with reference to two case-reports. Joint Bone Spine 2003;70:307–9.
5. Jahss ML. The sesamoids of the hallux. Clin Orthop Relat Res 1981;157:88–97.
6. Leventen EO. Sesamoid disorders and treatment. Clin Orthop 1991;269:236–40.
7. Sammarco HG. Dance injuries. Contemp Orthop 1984;8:15–27.
8. Jahss MS. Disorders of the foot and ankle: medical and surgical management. 2nd edition. Philadelphia: WB Saunders; 1991. p. 1062–75.
9. Kliman ME, Fross AE, Pritzker KP, et al. Osteochondritis of the hallux sesamoid bones. Foot Ankle 1983;3:220–3.
10. Karasick D. Disorders of the hallux sesamoid complex. Skeletal Radiol 1998;27:411–8.
11. Rath B, Notermans HP, Frank D, et al. Arterial anatomy of the hallucal sesamoids. Clin Anat 2009;22:755–60.
12. Pretterklieber ML. Dimensions and arterial vascular supply of the sesamoid bones of the human hallux. Acta Anat (Basel) 1990;139(1):86–90.
13. Pretterklieber M, Wanivenhaus A. The arterial supply of the sesamoid bones of the hallux: the course and source of the nutrient arteries as an anatomical basis for surgical approaches to the great toe. Foot Ankle 1992;13:27–31.
14. Chamberland PD, Smith JW, Fleming LL. The blood supply to the great toe sesamoids. Foot Ankle 1993;14(8):435–42.
15. Sobel M, Hashimoto J, Arnoczky S, et al. The microvasculature of the sesamoid complex: its clinical significance. Foot Ankle 1992;13:359 63.
16. Ogata K, Sugioka Y, Urano Y, et al. Idiopathic osteonecrosis of the first metatarsal sesamoid. Skeletal Radiol 1986;15(2):141–5.
17. Pinto RR, Freitas D, Massada M, et al. Hallux sesamoid osteonecrosis associated to ballet: literature review. Rev Port Ortop Traum 2010;18(4):429–37.
18. Waizy H, Jager M, Abbara-Czardybon M, et al. Surgical treatment of AVN of the fibular (lateral) sesamoid. Foot Ankle Int 2008;29(2):231–6.
19. Oloff LM, Schulhofer SD. Sesamoid complex disorders. Clin Podiatr Med Surg 1996;13:497–513.
20. Barral CM, Felix AM, Magalhaes LN, et al. The bone scintigraphy as a complementary exam in the diagnosis of the avascular necrosis of the sesamoid. Rev Bras Ortop 2012;47(2):241–5.
21. Richardson EG. Injuries to the hallucial sesamoids in the athlete. Foot Ankle 1987;7:229–44.
22. Julsrud M. Osteonecrosis of the tibial and fibular sesamoids in an aerobics instructor. J Foot Ankle Surg 1997;36:31–5.
23. Aper R, Saltzman C, Brown T. The effect of hallux sesamoid resection on the effective moment of the flexor hallucis brevis. Foot Ankle Int 1994;15:462–70.

24. Inge GAL, Ferguson AB. Surgery of the sesamoid bones of the great toe. Arch Surg 1933;27:466–88.
25. Mann RA, Coughlin MJ, Baxter D, et al. Sesamoidectomy of the great toe. Presented at the 15th Annual Meeting of the American Orthopaedic Foot and Ankle Society, Las Vegas, January 24, 1985.

Freiberg Disease and Avascular Necrosis of the Metatarsal Heads

Andrew Wax, BS[a], Robert Leland, MD[b],*

KEYWORDS

- MRI • Osteochondrosis • Radiograph • Weight-bearing

KEY POINTS

- Freiberg disease is an uncommon disease with variable presentations over a wide age range.
- Treatment options must take into consideration the patient's age, symptoms, stage of pathology, and overall foot mechanics.
- Despite significant radiographic findings, patients are often asymptomatic and require no treatment or modest nonsurgical management.
- When symptoms warrant, and surgery is proposed, there is no clear consensus based on a limited amount of studies which option is best.

INTRODUCTION

Dr Albert H Freiberg first described the so-called infraction, or avascular necrosis (AVN), of the second metatarsal head in 1914. As such, the disease was eponymously named. Freiberg noted 6 cases of female patients, either adolescent or younger than middle-aged. Clinically, his patients complained of pain overlying the ball of the foot associated with weight bearing. Radiographically, he defined a "crushed in" second metatarsal head and development of loose bodies within the second metatarsophalangeal (MTP) joint. Four of his patients were treated nonoperatively with rigid, mechanical support, whereas the remaining 2 ultimately required surgical intervention.[1]

Freiberg disease is characterized as osteochondrosis of the second metatarsal head. It is the fourth most common form of primary osteochondrosis with a significant predilection to the adolescent athletic female population, although it has been seen over a wide age range.[2–5] If treated early, osteochondroses such as Freiberg disease are essentially self-limiting, often resolving with nonoperative management.[6] When surgery is warranted, it is imperative the patient's age, activity level, and degree of articular deformity be taken into account.

The author has nothing to disclose.
[a] Boulder Centre for Orthopedics, 4740 Pearl Parkway, Boulder, CO 80301, USA; [b] Department of Orthopedic Surgery, University of Colorado School of Medicine, 12631 E. 17th Avenue, Aurora, CO 80045, USA
* Corresponding author.
E-mail address: rhleland@comcast.net

Foot Ankle Clin N Am 24 (2019) 69–82
https://doi.org/10.1016/j.fcl.2018.11.003
1083-7515/19/© 2018 Elsevier Inc. All rights reserved.

ETIOLOGY

It is generally accepted that the condition is of multifactorial cause, including trauma, foot mechanics, and arterial insufficiency.[3,7–10] There are several identified systemic risk factors for Freiberg disease, including hypercoagulability, systemic lupus erythematosus, and diabetes mellitus, but research surrounding these is sparse.[3,11,12] Furthermore, the disease is likely to have a genetic component, because there has been report of Freiberg disease and other osteochondroses in identical twins.[13,14] Despite all of this, cause surrounding Freiberg disease remains unclear.

Trauma and Abnormal Biomechanics

Rarely will a patient present with acute onset of pain secondary to a specific inciting injury. Rather, it is common for pain to have insidious and/or progressive onset. This is likely to be related to microtrauma in the form of minor repeat assault and/or abnormal weight bearing and gradual overload to dorsal aspect of the joint, causing undue trabecular stress at the epiphysis.[1,3,7,8,15,16]

Freiberg disease most often affects the second MTP joints and is less frequently observed at the third, fourth, and fifth MTP joints.[17] The second and third metatarsals are the longest and most susceptible to overload especially in the setting of an incompetent first ray.[18] The static articulation at the Lisfranc joints and inherent stability of the second metatarsal as the keystone of the foot further indicate its generalized susceptibility to overload and subsequent injury. Further exacerbating this factor, congenital gastrocnemius contracture is widely acknowledged as a noteworthy driving force for lesser metatarsal overload.[19]

Lastly, mechanical overload due to choice of shoe wear has been hypothesized as a potential risk factor. Specifically, the hyperdorsiflexed position associated with use of high-heeled shoes has been postulated to increase dorsal subchondral stress and may partially explain the female prevalence.[5] In collocation, foot pressure studies by Betts and colleagues[20] have shown that there is no significant overload at the infracted joints as compared with the unaffected population.

Arterial Insufficiency

It has been established that vascular flow to the lesser metatarsal heads is supplied by the dorsal metatarsal arteries and the plantar metatarsal arteries, which are a branch of the posterior tibial artery. It can be surmised that anatomic variants lacking a source of arterial flow are predisposed to ischemia, as shown by Wiley and Thurston in their cadaveric injection studies, whereby second metatarsals lacking normal arterial flow were instead supplied by collateral vessels from the first and third metatarsals.[21]

Although not proved, the aforementioned anatomic variants are likely to be susceptible to arterial congestion ancillary to inflammatory changes mediated by lesser metatarsal overload.[21,22] In the event of collateral arterial obstruction, Viladot and Viladot[23] theorized the following 5 stages of Freiberg disease as pathophysiologic explanation:

1. Mechanical arterial compression
2. Arterial spasm
3. Epiphyseal ischemia
4. Vascular occlusion
5. Bone resorption, remodeling, collapse, and eventual joint arthrosis

Clinical Presentation

As briefly discussed previously, Freiberg disease is likely to afflict women aged adolescent to those younger than middle-aged but may present in both men and women in a wide range of ages. The disease is most commonly observed overlying the second MTP joint (68% of cases) but has been known to affect the third MTP (27%), the fourth MTP (3%), and the fifth MTP (<2%).[17] Less than 10% of patients with Freiberg disease present with bilateral symptoms.[9]

Patients predominantly complain of pain overlying the plantar forefoot at the level of the second MTP joint (or other lesser MTP), exacerbated by walking barefoot or while wearing shoes with poor forefoot rigidity and/or elevated heel.

Physical examination likely reveals a joint effusion and exquisite plantar/dorsal tenderness directly overlying the affected joint. Other examination findings are likely to include diminished MTP range of motion with palpable crepitation and increased anterior laxity as compared with the opposite side. Silfverskiold test should be performed to assess gastrocnemius equinus, because certain surgical options may be predicated on this. Finally, advanced Freiberg disease may present with claw and/ or crossover toe deformity.[10]

Radiographic Evaluation

Radiographs
Anteroposterior, lateral, and oblique weight-bearing radiographs of the affected foot should be performed. Early radiographic evaluation of osteochondroses such as Freiberg disease is often unremarkable.[6] The earliest radiographic manifestation of Freiberg disease is observed approximately 3 to 6 weeks following initial onset of symptoms and are characterized as subtle joint space widening.[24] As the condition progresses, gradual collapse of the affected metatarsal head may be observed dorsally (**Fig. 1**).

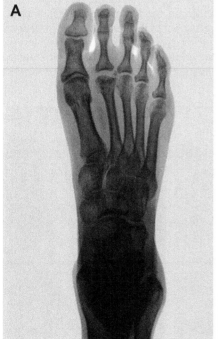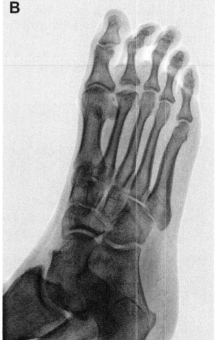

Fig. 1. Radiographs. (*A*) AP radiograph and (*B*) oblique radiograph. AP, anteroposterior.

MRI

MRI evaluation is important both from a staging standpoint as well as for preoperative planning. Before plain radiographic findings, early stage Freiberg disease may be apparent on MR images demonstrating increased marrow signal. Important factors include location of articular compromise, location of articular preservation, osseous defects, presence of intraarticular loose fragments and bone marrow edema. Preservation of more plantar articular cartilage is best assessed on the sagittal images, which is necessary if a rotational osteotomy is to be considered as a treatment option (**Fig. 2**).[7]

Classification and Staging

Gillespie (osteochondrosis progression)

Osteochondroses are a classification of epiphyseal disorders most commonly appreciated in the immature skeleton. Gillespie[4] established that osteochondroses follow a unique evolution. Initial osteochondral necrosis is followed by revascularization and reorganization with formation and invasion of granulation tissue. Subsequently, osteoclasts resorb necrotic portions and osteoid replacement of mature lamellar bone will occur. Freiberg disease, although distinctive, follows a similar progression, which has been previously and effectively described.

Smillie

Smillie[25] was the first to describe a system of staging based largely on surgical findings but is also applicable to radiographic appearance. Five stages were proposed (**Fig. 3**).

- The first stage represents the development of a chondral fissure overlying the epiphysis of a mildly osteopenic metatarsal head secondary to ischemia.
- The second stage is the earliest to be observed radiographically, demonstrating a mildly sunken appearance of the central aspect of the dorsum of the metatarsal head.
- The third stage shows a further sunken appearance overlying the metatarsal head due to gradual resorption. These findings are accompanied by subsequent

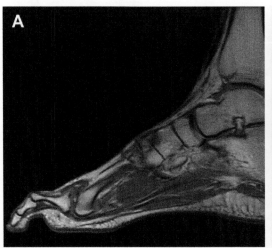
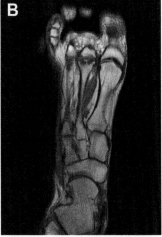

Fig. 2. MRI. (*A*) Sagittal T1 and (*B*) axial T1.

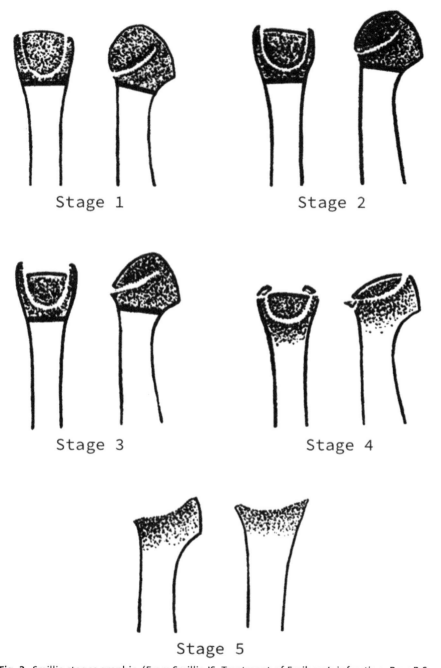

Stage 1   Stage 2

Stage 3   Stage 4

Stage 5

Fig. 3. Smillie stages graphic. (*From* Smillie IS. Treatment of Freiberg's infraction. Proc R Soc Med 1967;60(1):29–31; with permission.)

development of bony projections both medially and laterally. The plantar articular cartilage remains intact.

- During the fourth stage, the bony projections fracture, forming intraarticular loose bodies, and the plantar articular cartilage isthmus give way. Evolution at this point is incapable of anatomic restoration.
- Finally, the fifth stage is composed of joint arthrosis.

Gauthier and Elbaz

In a 1979 study of 88 surgical cases of Freiberg disease treated with metatarsal dorsiflexion osteotomy, Gauthier and Elbaz[17] developed 5 stages of anatomic evolution:

- Stage 0: subchondral bone march fracture in the setting of unremarkable radiographs; capable of consolidating
- Stage 1: osteonecrosis independent of deformation; capable of consolidating
- Stage 2: osteonecrosis with evidence of crushing deformation; capable of consolidating
- Stage 3: progressive chondral damage; irreparable
- Stage 4: arthrosis

Thompson and Hamilton

Finally, Thompson and Hamilton[26] similarly proposed a 4-type classification protocol for Freiberg disease with associated treatment recommendations.

- Type I Freiberg disease is more or less ephemeral in nature, impartial to any osteochondral damage. Nonoperative treatment is likely to be the mainstay.
- Type II involves a more impactful ischemic insult with development of periarticular spurring, yet articular cartilage remains intact. Overall clinical and radiographic pictures indicate MTP joint cheilectomy and debridement.
- Type III demonstrates severe degenerative joint disease with apparent loss of articular cartilage. A more invasive surgical approach is necessary, to comprise joint sacrificing procedures, as will be discussed later on.
- Type IV Freiberg disease is defined as epiphyseal dysplasia and is likely to involve multiple metatarsal heads. Treatment is predicated on the stage of the disease as previously outlined. Type IV is irrefutably rare.

TREATMENT FOR FREIBERG DISEASE
Nonoperative Management

Because these lesions are often asymptomatic or previously asymptomatic, the goal of nonoperative treatment is to achieve symptoms that are tolerable despite potentially significant pathology.

Shoe wear modifications

Standard shoe wear directed toward limiting forefoot motion, cushioning the impact at the MTP joints and providing a forefoot rocker can take the strain off the irritated second MTP joint. Although custom shoe modifications and inserts are available, typically an over-the-counter graphite foot plate and a commercially available shoe are equally successful at a significant cost saving (**Figs. 4** and **5**).

Steroid injections may be considered as a means of improving an acutely inflamed joint. As with most chronic degenerative conditions, this is unlikely to provide lasting relief but may be a temporizing measure. Concerns over repeated steroid injections exist.

Regenerative medicine injections including platelet-rich plasma, stem cell, amniotic tissue, and exosomes may have a role in reparation of the cartilage deficiency

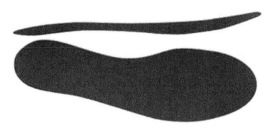

Fig. 4. Carbon fiber extended shank.

associated with Freiberg disease but will not address any bony deficiency or exostosis development associated with the condition. The use of these modalities is currently evolving. To date, there are no studies that have investigated the efficacy of these injections as a means of treating the osteocartilaginous defects associated with Freiberg disease.

Operative Management

Operative management of Freiberg osteonecrosis should be reserved for patients whose pain and functional limitations are unacceptable with nonsurgical management. Surgical treatment can be grouped into "joint preserving" and "joint sacrificing." When planning surgical options, consideration into joint deformity, length and mobility of the first ray, second metatarsal length, and other factors such as gastrocnemius contracture need to be factored into decision-making. Although a variety of options have been described, many with favorable results, most of the reports in the literature are either case reports or involve a limited number of patients. There is no clear consensus as to which option is best. It is prudent to thoroughly assess each patient and individualize the surgical option based on the severity of deformity, joint morphology, age, and functional demands.

Joint Preservation

Options for joint preservation include debridement, osteotomy, and cartilage replacement. These may be performed separately or in combination.

Debridement

Debridement alone is reserved for patients with pain stemming from bony impingement without a significant bone or cartilage defect or from intraarticular loose bodies.

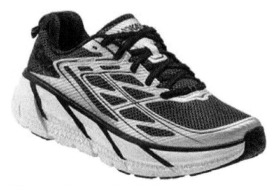

Fig. 5. Shoe with stiff sole, cushion, and forefoot rocker.

This is less likely to provide a favorable outcome in later stages of the disease. Both open and arthroscopic techniques are options. Open debridement is performed through a standard dorsal approach to the MTP joint. Although this may provide pain relief, it may be a temporizing measure because the cartilage deficit persists. Freiberg and others[1,25,27,28] have reported debridement of the joint with overall favorable results using both open and arthroscopic techniques (**Fig. 6**).

Osteotomies for Freiberg disease include rotational and shortening options. If the cartilage on the plantar aspect of the metatarsal head is relatively free of wear, rotation of the head via a dorsal closing wedge osteotomy can be performed. In cases where the second metatarsal is long leading to further overload at the second MTP joint, shortening the metatarsal at the same osteotomy site or proximally is recommended. Advantages of an osteotomy include maintenance of the patient's own tissue to restore a cartilage surface to the main articulating portion of the joint. In addition, mechanical overload from a long or plantarflexed second ray can be corrected. If failure occurs, the overall structural integrity is preserved, allowing for other reconstructive options. Like most osteotomies aimed at joint preservation, the articular surface remains compromised and may be a source of continued pain.

The dorsiflexion osteotomy has been described as either an intraarticular[17,29] or an extraarticular osteotomy.[30,31] Using a dorsal approach, an oblique dorsal closing wedge osteotomy directed in a dorsal distal to plantar proximal direction is used to orient the plantar cartilage into a position that articulates with the proximal phalanx. Various fixation methods have been proposed, but rigid screw fixation is preferable resulting in a stable construct that allows for immediate weight bearing and early joint

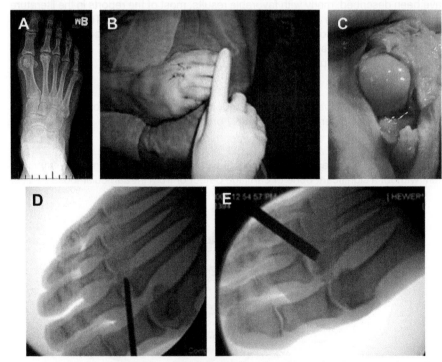

Fig. 6. Arthroscopic debridement. (*A*) Preoperative AP radiograph, (*B*) incisions for arthroscopic debridement, (*C*) intraoperative chondral damage, (*D*) arthroscopic evaluation, (*E*) arthroscopic debridement. (*Courtesy of* Alastair Younger, MD, Vancouver BC, Canada.)

mobilization. The intraarticular osteotomy first described in 1979 by Gauthier and Elbaz[17] produced favorable results in 52 out of 53 patients. Most recently, in 2016, Pereira and colleagues[32] showed very favorable long-term follow-up at a mean of 23.4 years (range 15–32 years) (**Fig. 7**).

Chondral Graft

Cartilage replacement can consist of autogenous osteochondral grafting, osteochondral allograft, or chondral allograft.

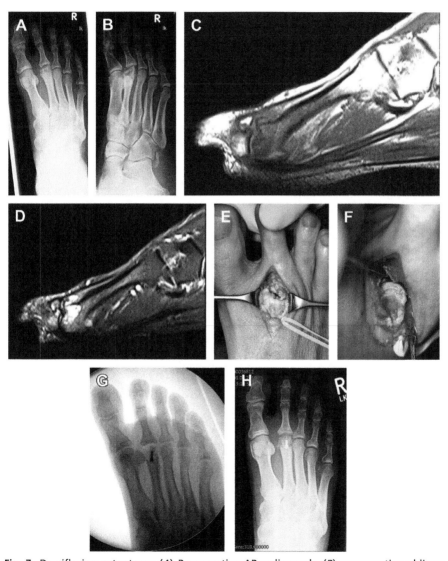

Fig. 7. Dorsiflexion osteotomy. (*A*) Preoperative AP radiograph, (*B*) preoperative oblique radiograph, (*C*) sagittal T1 MRI, (*D*) sagittal FS MRI, (*E*) intraoperative condition of the second metatarsal head, (*F*) intraoperative osteotomy, (*G*) intraoperative fluoroscopic image, (*H*) 2-year follow-up AP radiograph. FS, fat-saturation. (*Courtesy of* Stefan Rammelt, MD, Dresden, Germany.)

Much like in other joint surfaces with osteochondral deficiencies such as the femoral condyle or talus, osteochondral transplantation from the "less essential" portion of the distal femur can be used both to fill the osseous void associated with late-stage Freiberg disease and to replace the deficient joint cartilage. Advantages include a more viable, fresh source for chondrocyte transfer with predictable incorporation of the bone graft. Disadvantages include potential for host site morbidity and "mismatch" of the chondral surface due to the graft not perfectly replicating the exact contour of the second metatarsal head. Initially described by Hayashi and colleagues, additional reports, all with limited patient numbers, have shown favorable clinical and radiographic results.

Osteochondral allograft reconstruction can be used in a similar manner to autogenous grafting or as a joint salvage via a bulk allograft. Advantages include the potential to obtain a closely matched joint surface compared with the patient's normal anatomy, avoidance of potential harvest morbidity, and a readily accessible source. Disadvantages include concerns over viability of allograft chondrocytes and potential disease transmission. A limited series of 2 patients by Ajis and colleagues[33] showed favorable outcomes at final follow-up (**Fig. 8**).

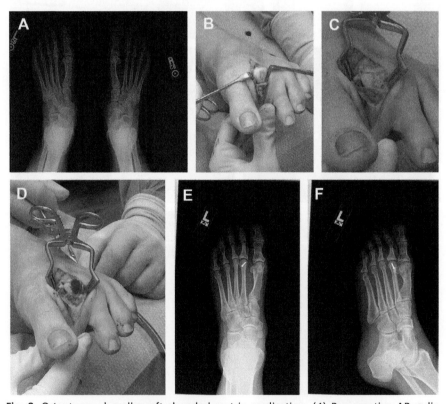

Fig. 8. Osteotomy plus allograft chondral matrix application. (*A*) Preoperative AP radiograph, (*B*) intraoperative condition of the second metatarsal head, (*C*) intraoperative image after osteotomy and preparation of the metatarsal head, (*D*) intraoperative after application of allograft matrix, (*E*) 2-year follow-up AP radiograph, (*F*) 2-year follow-up oblique radiograph. (*Courtesy of* Sarang Desai, DO, Frisco, TX.)

Chondrocyte Transfer

Use of juvenile chondrocyte transfer, as has been described for chondral defects in the femoral condyle and talus, has been described by Desai[34] in conjunction with an osteotomy as a means for restoring the articular deficiency associated with Freiberg disease. A standard dorsal incision is used for joint access. After removal of prominent osteophytes, the bone surface on the metatarsal head is prepared for transplant by creating a raw bone surface and drilling the subchondral surface multiple times with a small-diameter drill bit. The allograft cartilage matrix is applied and sealed with a fibrin gel. At 2-year follow-up, the patient in Desai's case report was pain free with radiographs showing a concentric metatarsal head.

Joint Sacrificing Procedures

Metatarsal head resection

Excision of the metatarsal head is mainly of historical significance. Although this operation may improve pain at the joint, the unacceptable amount of shortening caused predictably produces unacceptable long-term outcomes. Furthermore, excision of the head leaves any future reconstructive options extremely difficult.

Interpositional arthroplasty

Use of autogenous or allograft soft tissue grafts as a biological spacer have been described with favorable outcomes as a means of providing a "new" joint space to the diseased second MTP joint.[35–37] Using a standard dorsal approach, various tissues including the dorsal capsule, extensor digitorum longus, or extensor digitorum brevis have been used to create a space between the metatarsal head and the proximal phalanx. Allograft soft tissue grafts have the benefit of not limiting graft size but at a significantly increased price compared with autograft options. Advantages of

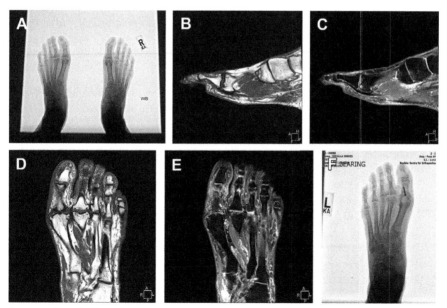

Fig. 9. Polyvinyl alcohol implant hemiarthroplasty. (*A*) Preoperative AP radiograph, (*B*) sagittal T1 MRI, (*C*) sagittal FS MRI, (*D*) coronal T1 MRI, (*E*) coronal FS MRI, (*F*) postoperative AP radiograph.

interpositional arthroplasty include the ability to create a space in the arthritic joint and allow for mobilization of the toe. Furthermore, if failure occurs, the procedure does not compromise any additional reconstructive options. The main disadvantage is lack of any long-term outcome studied showing that this will stand up over time.

Implant arthroplasty

Historically, silicone implants for lesser toe joint replacement have been used providing mixed short-term results and consistent long-term failure. Osteolysis, loosening, and synovitis usually lead to implant removal and the subsequent problems associated with a resection arthroplasty. Other materials such as titanium and ceramic have been used as a hemiarthroplasty in limited case studies with inconsistent results. Although the bone sacrifice associated with these implants is less compared with silicone, failure still presents a very difficult salvage. A newer "synthetic cartilage" (polyvinyl alcohol hydrogel) implant received approval from Food and Drug Administration in the United States after more than 5 years of use in Canada and Europe for operative treatment of first MTP arthrosis. Although currently not approved for lesser metatarsal use, the implant provides for a new "space" without sacrificing structural bone, should revision be necessary in the future (**Fig. 9**).

SUMMARY

Freiberg disease is an uncommon disease with variable presentations over a wide age range. Treatment options must take into consideration the patient's age, symptoms, stage of pathology, and overall foot mechanics. Despite significant radiographic findings, patients are often asymptomatic and require no treatment or modest nonsurgical management. When symptoms warrant, and surgery is proposed, there is no clear consensus based on a limited amount of studies which option is best. An individualized approach taking into consideration the degree of articular deformity is recommended. Based on the incidence of surgical procedures in patients in their second through fifth decades of life, it is imperative that any operative approach not compromise any future reconstructive efforts, should failure occur.

REFERENCES

1. Freiberg AH. Infraction of the second metatarsal bone: a typical injury. Surg Gynecol Obstet 1914;19:191–3.
2. Omer GE, Siffert RS. Primary articular osteochondroses. Clin Orthop Relat Res 1981;158:28–32.
3. Carmont MR, Rees RJ, Blundell CM. Current concepts review: Freiberg's disease. Foot Ankle Int 2009;30(2):167–76.
4. Gillespie H. Osteochondroses and apophyseal injuries of the foot in the young athlete. Curr Sports Med Rep 2010;9(5):265–8.
5. Katcherian DA. Treatment of Freiberg's disease. Orthop Clin North Am 1994; 25(1):69–81.
6. Danger F, Wasyliw C, Varich L. Osteochondroses. Semin Musculoskelet Radiol 2018;22(1):118–24.
7. Cerrato RA. Freiberg's disease. Foot Ankle Clin 2011;16(4):647–58.
8. Talusan PG, Diaz-Collado PJ, Reach JS. Freiberg's infraction: diagnosis and treatment. Foot Ankle Spec 2014;7(1):52–6.
9. Mandell GA, Harcke HT. Scintigraphic manifestations of infraction of the second metatarsal (Freiberg's disease). J Nucl Med 1987;28(2):249–51.

10. Seybold JD, Zide JR. Treatment of Freiberg disease. Foot Ankle Clin 2018;23(1): 157–69.

11. Nguyen VD, Keh RA, Daehler RW. Freiberg's disease in diabetes mellitus. Skeletal Radiol 1991;20(6):425–8.

12. Green N, Osmer JC. Small bone changes secondary to systemic lupus erythematosus. Radiology 1968;90:118–20.

13. Blitz NM, Yu JH. Freiberg's infraction in identical twins: a case report. J Foot Ankle Surg 2005;44(3):218–21.

14. Tsirikos AI, Riddle EC, Kruse RW. Bilateral Kohler's disease in identical twins. Clin Orthop Relat Res 2003;409:195–8.

15. Schade VL. Surgical management of Freiberg's infraction: a systematic review. Foot Ankle Spec 2015;8(6):498–519.

16. Freiberg AH. The so-called infraction of the second metatarsal bone. J Bone Jt Surgery1 1926;8(2):257–61.

17. Gauthier G, Elbaz R. Freiberg's infraction: a subchondral bone fatigue fracture. A new surgical treatment. Clin Orthop Relat Res 1979;142:93–5.

18. Bayliss NC, Klenerman L. Avascular necrosis of lesser metatarsal heads following forefoot surgery. Foot Ankle Int 1989;10(3):124–8.

19. Cortina RE, Morris BL, Vopat BG. Gastrocnemius recession for metatarsalgia. Foot Ankle Clin North Am 2018;23(1):57–68.

20. Betts RP, Stanley D, Smith TWD. Foot pressure studies in Freiberg's disease. Foot 1991;1(1):21–7.

21. Wiley JJ, Thurston P. Freiberg's disease. J Bone Jt Surg 1981;63:459.

22. Montgomery HC, Davies MB. Common disorders of the adult foot and ankle. Surg (United Kingdom) 2016;34(9):475–81.

23. Viladot A, Viladot A. Osteochondroses: aseptic necrosis of the foot. In: Disorders of the foot and ankle. 2nd edition. Philadelphia: Saunders; 1991. p. 617–38.

24. Hill J, Jimenez AL, Langford JH. Osteochondritis dissecans treated by joint replacement. J Am Podiatr Med Assoc 1979;69(9):556–61.

25. Smillie IS. Treatment of Freiberg's infraction. J R Soc Med 1967;60(1):29–31.

26. Thompson FM, Hamilton WG. Problems of the second metatarsophalangeal joint. Orthopedics 1987;10(1):83–9.

27. Sproul J, Klaaren H, Mannarino F. Surgical treatment of Freiberg's infraction in athletes. Am J Sports Med 1993;21(3):381–4.

28. Maresca G, Adriani E, Falez F, et al. Arthroscopic treatment of bilateral Freiberg's infraction. Arthrosc 1996;12(1):103–8.

29. Kinnard P, Lirette R. Dorsiflexion osteotomy in Freiberg's disease. Foot Ankle 1989;9(5):226–31.

30. Lee SK, Chung MS, Baek GH, et al. Treatment of Freiberg disease with intra-articular dorsal wedge osteotomy and absorbable pin fixation. Foot Ankle Int 2007;28(1):43–8.

31. Chao K-H, Lee C-H, Lin L, et al. Surgery for symptomatic Freiberg's disease Extraarticular dorsal closing-wedge osteotomy in 1 3 patients followed for 2-4 years. Acta Orthop Scand 1999;70(5):483–6.

32. Pereira BS, Frada T, Freitas D, et al. Long-term follow-up of dorsal wedge osteotomy for pediatric freiberg disease. Foot Ankle Int 2016;37(1):90–5.

33. Ajis A, Seybold JD, Myerson MS. Osteochondral distal metatarsal allograft reconstruction: a case series and surgical technique. Foot Ankle Int 2013;34(8): 1158–67.

34. Desai S. Freiberg's infarction treated with metatarsal shortening osteotomy, marrow stimulation, and micronized allograft cartilage matrix: a case report. Foot Ankle Spec 2017;10(3):258–62.
35. Özkan Y, Öztürk A, Özdemir R, et al. Interpositional arthroplasty with extensor digitorum brevis tendon in Freiberg's disease: a new surgical technique. Foot Ankle Int 2008;29(5):488–92.
36. Zgonis T, Jolly GP, Kanuck DM. Interpositional free tendon graft for lesser metatarsophalangeal joint arthropathy. J Foot Ankle Surg 2005;44(6):490–2.
37. Lui TH. Thompson and Hamilton type IV Freiberg's disease with involvement of multiple epiphyses of both feet. BMJ Case Rep 2015;2015 [pii:bcr2014206909].

Köhler Disease
Avascular Necrosis in the Child

Jeremy Y. Chan, MD[a], Jeffrey L. Young, MD[b],*

KEYWORDS

- Köhler disease • Navicular avascular necrosis • Pediatric patient • Midfoot pain

KEY POINTS

- Köhler disease refers to the condition of pain and swelling of the medial midfoot with associated osteochondrosis or avascular necrosis of the tarsal navicular in the child.
- Though the etiology of Köhler disease remains unknown and is likely multifactorial, the prevailing hypothesis suggests microtrauma to the cartilaginous navicular by the surrounding tarsal bones leads to disruption of the vascular supply of the bone.
- Long-term outcomes for Köhler disease is favorable regardless of the type of treatment, although a short period of immobilization with a short leg walking cast may reduce the duration of symptoms.

INTRODUCTION

Köhler disease refers to the condition of pain and swelling of the medial midfoot with associated osteochondrosis or avascular necrosis of the tarsal navicular in the child. Alban Köhler first described this condition in 1908[1], reporting on 3 children who presented with pain in the medial midfoot and radiographic abnormalities of the navicular. Unlike avascular necrosis of the navicular in adults, the condition in children is self-resolving. This article reviews the literature relevant to the etiology, diagnosis, and treatment of Köhler disease.

NAVICULAR ANATOMY AND ONTOGENESIS

The tarsal navicular occupies an important role in the midfoot serving as the primary bone that transmits body weight to the forefoot.[1] Rotation of the navicular around the talus allows for both adduction and abduction of the midfoot. Formed by the process of endochondral ossification, the navicular demonstrates significant variability in the timing and pattern of ossification. Ossification of the tarsal navicular occurs earlier in girls than boys. In girls, the tarsal navicular ossifies between the ages of 18 to 24 months; in comparison, ossification of the navicular occurs between 30 to

[a] Department of Orthopaedics, Stanford University, 300 Pasteur Drive, Edwards Building, R 144, Stanford, CA 94305-5341, USA; [b] Department of Orthopaedics, Stanford University, 300 Pasteur Drive, Edwards Building, R 105, Stanford, CA 94305-5341, USA
* Corresponding author.
E-mail address: jlyoung@stanford.edu

Foot Ankle Clin N Am 24 (2019) 83–88
https://doi.org/10.1016/j.fcl.2018.09.005
1083-7515/19/© 2018 Elsevier Inc. All rights reserved.

36 months in boys.[2,3] In regard to the ossification pattern, a review of radiographs for 100 randomly selected pediatric feet revealed that only two-thirds of tarsal naviculars develop from a single ossification center.[4] The remaining one-third of naviculars ossify from multiple centers. These patients with multiple ossification centers typically display a significant delay in the appearance of the navicular, consolidating at an average age of 5 to 6 years. In some cases, the heterogeneous radiographic appearance of the navicular from multiple overlapping ossification centers appears similar to the radiographic appearance of feet seen in patients with Köhler disease.

ETIOLOGY

The etiology of Köhler disease remains unknown. Early observers suggested an infectious insult as a cause, although laboratory values are usually within normal limits.[5] Others have proposed that Köhler disease represents a variation of normal development of the foot, as radiographic changes of the navicular are observed in asymptomatic feet.[6,7] A genetic predisposition for Köhler disease could be a possible contributing factor, as a case of bilateral Köhler disease has been reported in identical twins.[8] Meanwhile, there have been no associations found between Köhler disease and body weight or skeletal dysplasias.

The prevailing theory for Köhler disease focuses on the timing of ossification for the navicular and its potential role in the development of the condition. As the child begins early weight bearing, the navicular is subject to significant forces as the primary link between the talus and the forefoot. Due to its late ossification relative to the remaining tarsal bones, microtrauma to the largely cartilaginous navicular from surrounding structures could induce ischemia of the navicular through disruption of the arterial supply or venous congestion.[3] The navicular has been shown to be supplied by 1 or 2 main arterial branches from the dorsalis pedis and medial plantar artery, which anastomose into a perichondrial network surrounding the nonarticular surfaces of the bone.[3] These vascular channels could theoretically be disrupted with microtrauma, resulting in a compartment syndrome of the bone that could lead to the development of avascular necrosis. A similar phenomenon has been suggested to explain the development of avascular necrosis of the lunate in Keinbock disease.[9] Despite the hypothesized link to microtrauma of the navicular, reports of a specific antecedent trauma occurs in approximately one-third of patients with Köhler disease.[2]

DIAGNOSIS
Clinical Presentation

Children with Köhler disease present with variable symptoms, which may include pain and swelling localized to the navicular, as well as limping and a reluctance to apply pressure to the medial foot. Patients may relate symptoms to an injury such as a minor trauma, but in many instances, no specific event is recalled. Typically, the condition is unilateral but in approximately 15% to 20% of cases there is bilateral involvement.[2,10]

The usual child with this condition is a boy between the ages of 2 and 10 years.[2,7,10,11] Köhler disease occurs between 2 to 6 times more commonly in boys than girls.[2,3,7,10–12] As with the timing of ossification for the navicular, Köhler disease tends to occur at an earlier age in female patients compared with male patients. In girls, the average age at presentation is 3.5 to 4.5 years, whereas in boys, the average age at presentation is 5 to 6 years.[3,10] Development of avascular necrosis of the navicular in adolescence or adulthood is termed Brailsford disease or Mueller-Weiss syndrome, which is a distinct clinical entity from Köhler disease.[13,14]

Radiographic Findings

Initial imaging for patients suspected of Köhler disease should include weight-bearing radiographs of the foot. In a series of 62 children with Köhler disease, Waugh[3] described 2 distinct patterns in the appearance of the navicular. The more common pattern involves flattening of the navicular, often described as "waferlike," with patchy areas of sclerosis and loss of the normal bony trabecular architecture (**Fig. 1**). The second pattern involves uniform sclerosis of the navicular with maintenance of the overall shape. It has been hypothesized that the radiographic appearance of the navicular in Köhler disease is likely dependent on the source of its blood supply.[3] In the first pattern, patchy areas of sclerosis may indicate incomplete ischemia due to the presence of multiple arteries supplying the bone. When vascular supply originates from only a single vessel, a more uniform ischemia occurs resulting in the second radiographic pattern. Given that the normal ossification pattern of the tarsal navicular can produce radiographic findings seen in patients with Köhler disease, it is important to emphasize that the diagnosis of Köhler disease is dependent on the presence of clinical symptoms.

There are limited indications for more advanced forms of imaging, such as computed tomography (CT) or MRI, in the management of Köhler disease, as the additional information rarely results in a change in treatment plan. In cases in which the underlying diagnosis is unclear, CT or MRI may be useful to rule out other pathologies such as inflammatory arthritis, infection, or tarsal coalitions. In Köhler disease, MRI will generally demonstrate low signal intensity in the navicular on T1-weighted sequences and high intensity on T2-weighted images consistent with avascular necrosis. Some investigators have advocated for the role of bone scintigraphy to aid in diagnosis during the early stages of Köhler disease, when radiographs may appear normal.[15,16] On scintigraphy, the navicular will show decreased uptake on both dynamic and static images suggestive of reduced blood flow. Subsequent reimaging demonstrates restoration of uptake indicating revascularization of the navicular.

Differential Diagnosis

The differential diagnosis for Köhler disease includes inflammatory arthritis, posterior tibial tendonitis, tarsal coalition, accessory navicular, and infection. Unlike Köhler disease, patients with inflammatory arthritis experience pain in the surrounding tarsal joints, including pain with range of motion of the subtalar and tibiotalar joints. Patients with posterior tibial tendonitis often note pain in the medial midfoot and may have a planovalgus foot deformity. A tarsal coalition may present similarly. However, these

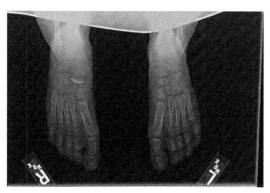

Fig. 1. Radiographic imaging of bilateral feet in a child with right foot pain. The radiograph demonstrates flattening and sclerosis of the navicular consistent with Köhler disease.

conditions usually occur in early adolescence and seldom show the radiographic findings seen in Köhler disease. In the cases of a tarsal coalition or an accessory navicular, radiographic findings correlate to their respective diagnosis. Finally, infection such as septic arthritis or osteomyelitis can present with pain, swelling, and a limp as well. These symptoms will likely be associated with laboratory abnormalities that are usually not seen with Köhler disease.

CLINICAL MANAGEMENT
Nonoperative Management

Management of Köhler disease is nonoperative. Mildly symptomatic feet have been managed with a variety of interventions, including rigid sole shoes, arch supports, non–weight bearing with crutches, and casting. Retrospective studies noted trends to earlier resolution of symptoms with immobilization in a weight-bearing short leg cast compared with alternative treatments.[10,12] Williams and Cowell[10] reported resolution of symptoms of 3.2 months for patients managed in a cast, versus 15.2 months in patients managed without casting. Those patients who underwent cast immobilization of more than 8 weeks seemed to have the shortest duration of symptoms, with an average of 2.5 months. Similar findings have been reported by Ippolito and colleagues,[12] who noted that patients immobilized with a cast for 3 months had resolution of symptoms on cast removal.

At our institution, management of Köhler disease varies by the severity of a patient's symptoms. When the pain is mild, we generally recommend use of a CAM boot for protection and use of crutches while allowing weight bearing as tolerated. A short leg cast is also offered, but generally only to patients with more severe symptoms who have difficulty weight bearing elect this option. Casting is seldom continued beyond 6 weeks because of concerns of foot stiffness from prolonged immobilization. Nonsteroidal anti-inflammatory medications may decrease pain symptoms. Patients are followed until symptoms resolve, with serial radiographic imaging of symptomatic feet. Images are reviewed to verify that no other diagnosis should be considered. If symptoms are worsening or pain is more than mild by 3 months, then advanced imaging, such as MRI, is considered to identify other causes for pain.

Operative Management

Longitudinal studies of Köhler disease have consistently demonstrated resolution of symptoms in all patients who undergo nonoperative management.[2,10–12] As a result, there are no reported cases in the literature that describe the use of operative treatment in the acute management of Köhler disease. In patients with recalcitrant symptoms despite multiple rounds of cast immobilization and rest, additional investigation is warranted to identify alternative causes for pain, such as the presence of a tarsal coalition or accessory navicular.[11]

PROGNOSIS

The overall prognosis for patients with Köhler disease is favorable. Long-term studies have shown little to no sequelae of Köhler disease. Radiographically, there is restoration of the navicular to near-normal anatomy at an average of 2 to 3 years[2,3] (**Fig. 2**). Notably, the treatment technique does not appear to affect the time until radiographic improvement.[2] From a clinical perspective, Williams and Cowell[10] published a case series of 20 patients with an average of 10-year follow-up, and all patients were asymptomatic and without radiographic evidence of osteoarthritis. Ippolito and colleagues[12] reported on 30-year to 37-year follow-up, with all 12 patients having

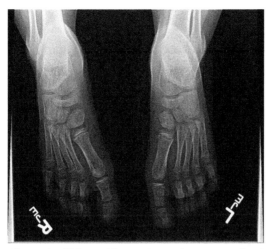

Fig. 2. Follow-up radiograph of bilateral feet at 1 year shows normalization of the navicular, with slight residual narrowing of the space between the medial cuneiform and the talus.

resolution of symptoms and no recurrence of pain. Imaging of the affected extremity showed no degenerative changes. Borges and colleagues[11] reported 24-year to 44-year follow-up of 16 patients, similarly reporting outcomes of no pain, good motion, ability to participate in sports, and no limitations in walking distances in all but 2 patients. One of those 2 patients had a talocalcaneal coalition, whereas the other had an accessory navicular. The development of a talonavicular coalition has been reported following Köhler disease.[17] In this case report, the patient was noted to develop a lateral talonavicular bar on radiograph during reossification of the navicular, which subsequently became symptomatic at 10 years of age. The coalition was successfully treated with a period of immobilization without the need for operative intervention.

SUMMARY

Köhler disease is defined by the development of avascular necrosis of the navicular in children. The diagnosis is based on symptoms such as pain, swelling, and a limp in association with characteristic radiographic findings of sclerosis, flattening, and fragmentation of the navicular. Generally, this condition affects male patients younger than 10 years. When female patients are affected, symptoms tend to have an earlier onset. The evidence published to date regarding the etiology and treatment of Köhler disease is almost entirely based on multiple case series. Nevertheless, favorable outcomes following nonoperative management supports this approach to Köhler disease. Casting may lead to earlier resolution of symptoms, although long-term follow-up has demonstrated a favorable prognosis regardless of treatment. Further studies are needed to elucidate the underlying mechanisms behind the development of Köhler disease, which remains uncertain.

ACKNOWLEDGMENTS

The representative case was identified using STRIDE.[18]

REFERENCES

1. Köhler A. Ueber eine häufige, bisher anscheinend unbekannte Erkrankung einzelner kindlicher Knochen. MWW 1908;55:1923–5.

2. Karp MG. Köhler's disease of the tarsal scaphoid: an end-result study. JBJS 1937;19(1):84–96.
3. Waugh W. The ossification and vascularisation of the tarsal navicular and their relation to Köhler's disease. J Bone Joint Surg Br 1958;40-B(4):765–77.
4. Ferguson AB, Gingrich RM. The normal and abnormal calcaneal apophysis and tarsal navicular. Clin Orthop 1957;10:87–95.
5. Kidner FC, Muro F. Köhler's disease of the tarsal scaphoid or os naviculare pedis retardatum. JAMA 1924;83(21):1650–4.
6. Brower AC. The osteochondroses. Orthop Clin North Am 1983;14(1):99–117.
7. Viladot A, Rochera R, Viladot A. Necrosis of the navicular bone. Bull Hosp Jt Dis Orthop Inst 1987;47(2):285–93.
8. Tsirikos AI, Riddle EC, Kruse R. Bilateral Köhler's disease in identical twins. Clin Orthop Relat Res 2003;(409):195–8.
9. Bain GI, MacLean SBM, Yeo CJ, et al. The etiology and pathogenesis of Kienböck disease. J Wrist Surg 2016;5(4):248–54.
10. Williams GA, Cowell HR. Köhler's disease of the tarsal navicular. Clin Orthop Relat Res 1981;(158):53–8.
11. Borges JL, Guille JT, Bowen JR. Köhler's bone disease of the tarsal navicular. J Pediatr Orthop 1995;15(5):596–8.
12. Ippolito E, Ricciardi Pollini PT, Falez' F. Köhler's disease of the tarsal navicular: long-term follow-up of 12 cases. J Pediatr Orthop 1984;4(4):416–7.
13. Brailsford JF. Osteochondritis of the adult tarsal navicular. J Bone Joint Surg 1939;21(1):111–20.
14. Mohiuddin T, Jennison T, Damany D. Müller–Weiss disease. Review of current knowledge. Foot Ankle Surg 2014;20(2):79–84.
15. McCauley RG, Kahn PC. Osteochondritis of the tarsal navicula: radioisotopic appearances. Radiology 1977;123(3):705–6.
16. Khoury J, Jerushalmi J, Loberant N, et al. Kohler disease: diagnoses and assessment by bone scintigraphy. Clin Nucl Med 2007;32(3):179–81.
17. Ertel AN, O'Connell FD. Talonavicular coalition following avascular necrosis of the tarsal navicular. J Pediatr Orthop 1984;4(4):482–4.
18. Lowe HJ, Ferris TA, Hernandez PM, et al. STRIDE—an integrated standards-based translational research informatics platform. AMIA Annu Symp Proc 2009; 2009:391–5.

Management of Müller-Weiss Disease

Manuel Monteagudo, MD[a],*, Ernesto Maceira, MD[b]

KEYWORDS

- Müller-Weiss disease • Tarsal navicular • Avascular necrosis • Varus hindfoot
- Paradoxic planovarus • Calcaneal osteotomy

KEY POINTS

- Müller-Weiss disease (MWD) is a dysplasia of the tarsal navicular that is developed during childhood and suffered during adulthood.
- Pathomechanics in MWD include the shifting of the talar head laterally over the os calcis, thus driving the subtalar joint into varus.
- Failure to identify patients with paradoxic flatfeet (with hindfoot varus instead of conventional valgus) may lead to incorrect diagnosis and management.
- Conservative treatment with the use of rigid insoles with medial arch support and a lateral heel wedge to reduce supination of the heel is effective in most patients.
- Dwyer calcaneal osteotomy combined with lateral displacement seems to be a satisfactory treatment for the management of patients with MWD that had failed to respond to conservative measures. Joint-preserving surgery seems a good alternative to the different types of perinavicular fusions that do not address pathomechanics of MWD.

INTRODUCTION

Müller-Weiss disease (MWD) is an apparently uncommon finding in orthopedic daily practice. However, in the authors' experience, MWD is more common than might be expected. Failure to identify patients with paradoxic flatfeet (with hindfoot varus instead of conventional valgus) may lead to the incorrect diagnosis and management. Although there is no pathologic evidence of necrosis in most MWD patients, it has been largely considered to be an avascular necrosis of the tarsal navicular.

Delayed ossification of the tarsal navicular in young patients with a short first metatarsal allows for compressive forces to act on the lateral aspect of the bone, inducing

The authors have nothing to disclose.

[a] Orthopaedic Foot and Ankle Unit, Orthopaedic and Trauma Department, Hospital Universitario Quirónsalud Madrid, Calle Diego de Velazquez 1, UEM Madrid, Madrid 28223, Spain; [b] Orthopaedic and Trauma Department, Complejo Hospitalario La Mancha Centro, Alcázar de San Juan, Avenida Constitucion 3, Ciudad Real 13600, Spain
* Corresponding author.
E-mail address: mmontyr@yahoo.com

early dysplasia with flattening and fragmentation of the lateral one-third of the navicular. A short first metatarsal may fail to assume compressive stress during the third rocker of gait, thus resulting in shearing forces acting between the second ray (and lateral cuneiforms) and the talar head. These abnormal forces would increase deformity and eventual fragmentation of the cartilaginous navicular. The talar head would then move laterally and inferiorly following the flattening of the plantolateral aspect of the navicular. Pathomechanics in MWD include the shifting of the talar head laterally over the os calcis, thus driving the subtalar joint into varus. Equinization of the hindfoot takes place if enough space is available for the talar head to plantarflex, despite the fact that the calcaneus remains in an inverted position and the plantar soft tissues are not stretched; this produces a paradoxic "pes planus varus" with a prominent navicular in the medial aspect of the foot.

This review focuses on MWD and provides a basic understanding of the pathomechanics, clinical examination, and diagnostic studies. It fundamentally addresses the options for both conservative and surgical treatment of this challenging condition.

EPIDEMIOLOGY

Walther Müller and Konrad Weiss described a deforming condition of the navicular bone after the First World War (1914–1919).[1,2] In 1927, Müller was a German surgeon that published the first images of a compressed, condensed, and fragmented tarsal navicular. In 1925, Schmidt had already reported a similar affection in a patient with a multiple endocrine deficiency syndrome but showed no images.[1]

MWD is a navicular dysplasia that is almost always developed during childhood and suffered during adulthood. Deformity of the navicular with signs of compression, condensation, and fragmentation led Konrad Weiss (Austrian radiologist, and fellow of Kiemböck who had just described lunatomalacia) to believe that MWD was an osteonecrosis.[2] However, over the years, osteonecrotic changes have not been found in histologic studies except for isolated fragments or in cases with other concomitant conditions.[3–9] Perinavicular arthritis has been the main feature for most studies, but clinical symptoms may be attributed to the main pathomechanical change, which is present in all MWD cases: hindfoot varus. Most MWD patients also present with a short first metatarsal (index minus).

In a seminal paper on MWD, Maceira and Rochera[10] studied patients' records at Hospital San Rafael in Barcelona, Spain and found that 85% of patients with MWD had moved from rural areas in the south of Spain to live in Barcelona in the 1950s. Around 70% of patients (controls) attended at the same hospital at the same time for different conditions other than MWD were born in Barcelona. Most of the patients with MWD were immigrants whose families had moved to Barcelona escaping from hunger in southern Spain after the Spanish Civil War (1936–1939). A sudden onset of MWD cases was registered in the late 1920s, with a peak annual incidence in 1932. A second, smaller burst of MWD was noticed in 1948, just before the massive migratory movements from rural to urban areas that took place around the middle of the twentieth century in Spain. Under normal circumstances, ossification of the tarsal navicular initiates around 1.5 years of age in girls and 2 years of age in boys. Children had to undergo ossification of their navicular bones under severe environmental conditions at that time. It was clear that nutritional-environmental stress might have played a role in the pathogenesis of MWD. Those factors predisposing to the disease were also present in Europe (First and Second World Wars) but not in the United States. That difference might account for most of the reports and papers on MWD coming from Europe.

Delayed ossification of the navicular may be present as a localized or as a generalized developmental disturbance. Nutritional stress among children is known to be associated with Harris lines, dental enamel hypoplasia, and criba orbitalia. These findings are common in patients with MWD.

Apart from the clusters of cases, there are scattered cases with no environmental predisposing factors but who suffered conditions that affected growth of the tarsal navicular alone or the whole individual. Localized delayed ossification of the navicular may also be related to metatarsus adductus and clubfoot deformities and clubfoot deformities under the same pathomechanical setting.[10] In isolated cases, no predisposing factors have been found. Nowadays, the authors occasionally attend patients from the epidemic group, but most new MWD cases did not suffer from nutritional-environmental stress. From an epidemiologic point of view, the authors have identified 6 different settings that might influence the development of MWD:

1. Environmental epidemic stress during childhood
2. Nutritional individual stress during childhood
3. Obvious or subtle deformities comprising metatarsus adductus and hindfoot varus
4. Athletes with intensive training during childhood
5. Unknown origin
6. An adult-onset MWD that causes what is known as a "Müllerweissoid foot"

In a smaller group of patients, the authors have found evidence of a normal development of the navicular (eg, normal radiographs as young adults) that is later in life affected by associated mechanical conditions (subtalar varus, first ray brachymetatarsia, congenital or acquired, residual mild clubfoot) resulting in a similar presentation as MWD. "Müllerweissoid feet" are of special clinical relevance because they may be mistaken for acquired flatfeet, but tarsal deformity in these patients is just the opposite.[10]

PATHOMECHANICS

Is delayed ossification of the navicular alone enough for an MWD to develop? Surely not. There is most likely an abnormal force distribution pattern acting on the navicular to produce the characteristic asymmetrical compression of the lateral aspect of the bone. If compressive forces were homogeneously distributed across the entire tarsal navicular, the chondral anlage would possibly accommodate for them and no deformity would develop except for an eventual symmetric flattening in its anteroposterior width. Homogeneous distribution of compressive forces across the navicular possibly occur in Köhler disease, which is a self-limited benign condition, also known as *naviculare pedis retardatum*.

Three different pathogenic pathways may be present in MWD patients:

a. The so-called *epidemic group* with previous environmental/nutritional stress would include cases described by Müller, Weiss, de Fine Licht, Simons, Brailsford, and other authors.[1,2,7,11–14] "Children of war" were not able to sufficiently ossify their navicular bones. An immature (chondral) tarsal navicular would cope with compression stress as long as it is evenly distributed along its entire articular surface and the child has limited physical activities, even in the presence of delayed ossification (*navicularis pedis retardatum*).[15] It is necessary that a mechanical impairment producing lateral displacement of the compression stress acts on an immature navicular during a certain period of time for the chondral anlage to undergo plastic deformation. This deformation would be the result of shearing forces acting between the talar head and the lateral cuneiforms (**Fig. 1**). Primary subtalar

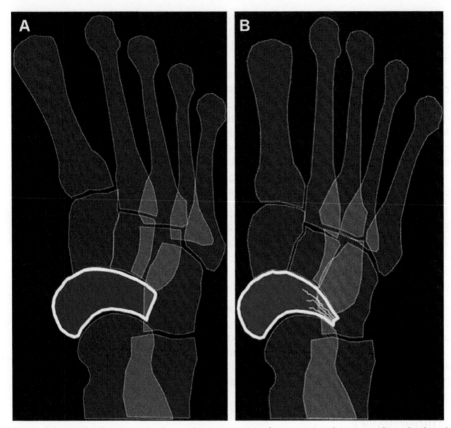

Fig. 1. (*A*) Nondysplastic navicular with compression forces acting between the talar head and the medial cuneiform. (*B*) Dysplastic navicular in MWD as a result of shearing forces acting between the talar head and the lateral navicular.

varus and first ray brachymetatarsia (index minus) would produce lateral transfer of compressive stress through the acetabulum pedis during the third rocker of the gait cycle, with the second and third rays assuming most of the axial stress. As deformation progresses, compressive forces would transform into shearing forces around the lateral aspect of the bone (**Fig. 2**). Some MWD patients show signs of subtle clubfeet. Fernández de Retana[16] studied a 4-year-old girl with a traumatic epiphysiodesis of the base of the first metatarsal that resulted in shortening of the first ray and later developed MWD.

b. The "*nonepidemic*" cases of MWD would not show criba orbitalia or other signs of environmental/nutritional stress (dental). In the authors' practice, they have noticed these patients are usually athletes who suffered intensive training during childhood ("too much too soon" for the navicular) affecting their navicular bones (even though they experienced the correct ossification schedule). Most of these children have a short first ray, either because of a short first metatarsal or as a result of a relative shortening of the medial column secondary to the internal rotation of the navicular on the transverse plane and relative retroposition of the first cuneometatarsal joint with respect to the second.[10] What would happen to a navicular of a child coping with mechanical stress more typical of an adult? It would possibly need a subtle

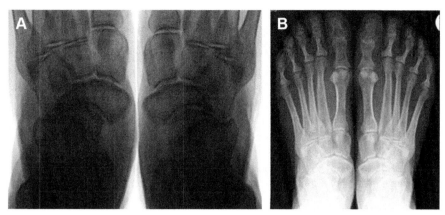

Fig. 2. (*A*) Bilateral MWD with talar heads shifting toward the lateral aspect of the naviculars. (*B*) Note index minus/short first metatarsal is present as a potential mechanical impairment.

alteration in mechanical load distribution (metatarsus adductus, primary or as a result of a subtle clubfoot, or subtalar varus or both) to produce the shifting of the talar head toward the lateral side of the coxa pedis (**Fig. 3**). Kidner and Muro[15] noticed that children with an adduction of the metatarsal palette showed a delayed ossification of their navicular bones. Spontaneous correction of the medial deviation of the forefoot may be observed when the cuneiforms and cuboid externally rotate "in-block." This rotation is possible if the medial aspect of the tarsal navicular is referenced as a fulcrum, thus rotating at the expense of the compression of the lateral aspect of the navicular and a medial subluxation of the cuboid. It would simulate a "nutcracker mechanism" with the arms being the talus and the cuneiforms, the fulcrum being the medial aspect of the navicular, and the nut being the lateral aspect of the navicular.

c. There is a third scenario in which the disease takes over an adult healthy navicular. The combined presence of subtalar varus and a short first metatarsal stimulates pronation of the forefoot with an arthritic Lisfranc joint. Lisfranc arthritis is evident, and midfoot abduction and pronation create a considerable dorsomedial prominence in the dorsal aspect of the midfoot ("dorsal beak") and false appearance of a flatfoot

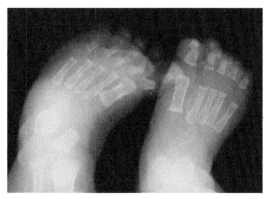

Fig. 3. Clubfoot deformity or metatarsus adductus may cause lateral displacement of the compression acting on an immature navicular.

with posterior tibialis dysfunction. However, one should beware that there is a subtalar joint varus and the talar head is damaging the lateral aspect of the acetabulum pedis. Lisfranc joint arthritis may draw attention away from the lateral talonavicular subluxation (**Fig. 4**). These "Müllerweissoid feet" may not show lateral navicular fragmentation but share pathomechanics with MWD and commonly present with arthrosis.[10] Some of these "Müllerweissoid feet" may end up developing a dysplasia of the navicular in which would be an adult-onset MWD.

CLINICAL EXAMINATION

Patients usually present with chronic pain on the dorsum of the foot and perinavicular pain around the fourth to fifth decades of life. Patients often complain of functional lateral ankle instability and refer pain around the peroneal tendons. Clinical examination may show a normal, high-, or low-arched foot with hindfoot varus. Varus can be subtle and only noticed on palpation of the heel during heel rise.

Clinical findings are variable, from patients suffering from a crippling condition due to perinavicular pain to almost asymptomatic patients showing advanced deformities. Apparently there is no direct correlation between navicular/foot deformity and pain. In most cases, patients with MWD seek attention for mechanical pain that was present for years before symptomatic worsening. Knee pain is common in MWD patients showing different degrees of knee osteoarthritis. It is common to find that some MWD patients have already undergone total knee replacement. Athletes with MWD suffer from knee pain without local pathologic radiographic changes in their knees. The authors believe knee pain is secondary to impaired mechanics of the whole limb rather than primary changes at the knee. Subtalar varus eliminates subtalar cushioning and midfoot compensation in the sagittal plane. Subtalar varus may explain knee pain as a result of the lack of cushioning at heel strike forcing the extensor mechanism of the knee to compensate for that rigid joint on every single step. External rotation of the leg may also cause femoropatellar maltracking and pain.

Regardless of the morphotype of the foot, patients with MWD show hindfoot varus deformity, which is present in all cases. Prominence of the medial aspect of the

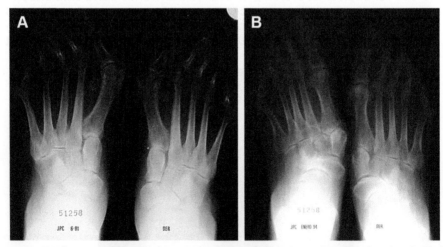

Fig. 4. "Müllerwessoid foot." (*A*) Dorsoplantar weight-bearing radiograph showing signs of subtle navicular dysplasia and index minus in 1981. (*B*) Same patient in 1994 with changes that demonstrate an adult-onset MWD.

navicular may give the false appearance of a flatfoot valgus deformity so palpation on heel raise and on subtalar movement is sometimes necessary to suspect MWD. In a flatfoot valgus deformity, the medial prominence is due to the talus, whereas in a paradoxic flatfoot varus in MWD, the medial prominence is due to the medially extruded navicular (talar head is shifted to plantar lateral) (**Fig. 5**). The leg is internally rotated in a flatfoot valgus, whereas it is externally rotated over the flatfoot varus in MWD. Paradoxic flatfoot varus deformities may also be noticed in some neurologic conditions, in residual clubfeet, after some navicular fractures, and so forth.

IMAGE AND OTHER DIAGNOSTIC STUDIES

Plain weight-bearing radiographs of both feet are necessary for the diagnosis and staging of MWD. Staging does not always correlate with the degree of pain and disability.[10] Many of the radiographic features are classic references for subtalar joint inversion. Image studies may help to understand mechanical impairments contributing to the typical navicular dysplasia. Plain weight-bearing radiographs may also help with the differential diagnosis between MWD and stress fractures of the navicular or with other types of talonavicular arthritis (rheumatoid, posttraumatic).[17,18]

What Does Tarsal Navicular in Müller-Weiss Disease Looks like in a Conventional Radiograph?

The *lateral weight-bearing view* shows reduction in the anteroposterior width of the tarsal navicular. Around half of the patients with MWD present with fragmentation and even splitting with an inclination from dorsal-distal to plantar-proximal or with a separate small dorsal fragment. Splitting is more commonly observed in the "epidemic group." There is an increased dorsoplantar length of the navicular as a result of the squeezing of the bone between the lateral cuneiforms and the talar head. Condensation is frequently present, although it is sometimes the result of superposition of the radiograph contours of the talar head and the navicular. Degenerative changes at

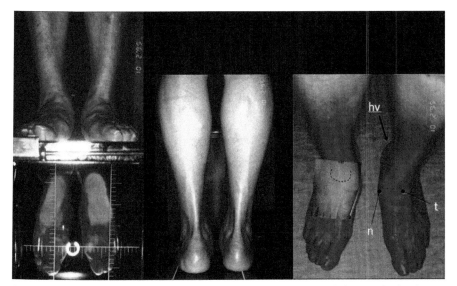

Fig. 5. Clinical presentation of MWD with paradoxic flatfoot varus deformity. hv, heel varus; n, navicular; t, talus.

the perinavicular joints are a common finding (**Fig. 6**). The lateral weight-bearing view allows classifying morphologic changes into 5 stages with increasing deformity in the sagittal plane (Maceira's classification), from minimal changes (stage 1) to advanced changes with extrusion of the navicular and talocuneiform contact (stage 5) (**Fig. 7**).[10] This classification has no prognostic value but provides valuable information to understand pathomechanics of MWD, especially in cases with subtle radiographic changes. Most MWD patients show bilateral affection with different radiographic stages. Subtalar varus deformity is inherent to MWD. On the lateral view, regardless of morphotype of the longitudinal arch, one may identify classic markers for subtalar joint varus: orthogonal projection of the subtalar, wide open sinus tarsi, increased retroposition of the fibula with respect to the tibia (external rotation of the leg with respect to the foot), reduced or no overlapping between talar head and anterior process of the os calcis, and the talar head placed beside and not over the anterior apophysis of the calcaneus.

The *dorsoplantar weight-bearing view* (**Fig. 8**) shows navicular deformity with variable degrees of compression. In advanced stages, the bone is compressed at its lateral aspect and presents a comma or hourglass shape. Fragmentation may be present with a medial hyperplasic portion of the bone, and a separated lateral portion is sometimes difficult to distinguish from the underlying cuboid. There is a systematic reduction of the talocalcaneal divergence (Kyte) indicating the existence of subtalar inversion/varus. The talar head moves laterally and is located over the anterior process of the calcaneus (instead of being by its medial side). The contour of the Chopart joint line resembles a "question mark" sign rather than the typical small "v" found between the 2 bones.[10] Several cases of MWD present with medial subluxation of the cuboid with respect to the calcaneus mimicking the cuboid sign described for clubfoot. There is a low incidence of hallux valgus, and index minus is a common finding on the dorsoplantar view (see **Fig. 8**). Index plus is only present in 1% of MWD patients.[10] Metatarsals are usually parallel to each other. Cuneiform-metatarsal joints are frequently externally rotated so that the first cuneiform-metatarsal joint tends to be perpendicular to the longitudinal axis of the foot and the second and third cuneiform-metatarsal joints are oriented laterally.

MRI and computed tomography will be of use for evaluation of fragmentation, bone stock, and extent of arthrosis, but are not usually essential.[19] The use of weight-bearing computed tomography scan is of interest to understand subtalar varus in MWD.[20] Plantar pressure studies have shown higher values at the midfoot combined with reduction in toe pressures and suggest hindfoot varus is an important feature in

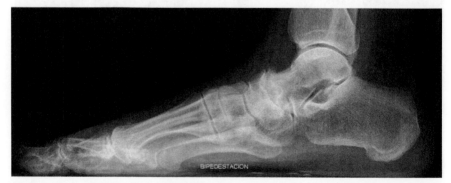

Fig. 6. Lateral weight-bearing radiograph showing an increase dorsoplantar length of the navicular, with condensation and degenerative changes at the talonavicular joint.

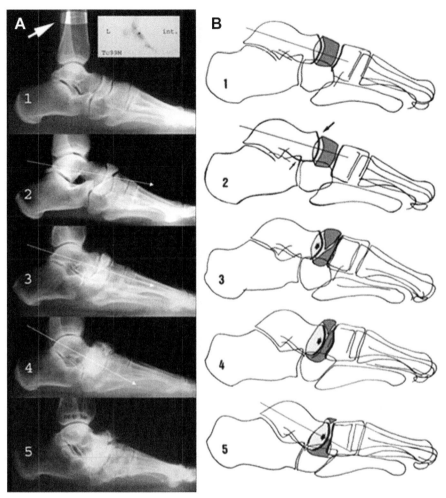

Fig. 7. Maceira's classification of MWD. (*A*) Schematic representation of the 5 stages with increasing deformity on the sagittal plane. Stage 1: minimal changes, Harris lines in distal tibia (*arrow*); stages 2 to 4: Orthogonal projection of the subtalar joint with the talar head lying over the anterior process of the calcaneus; stage 5: "talocuneiform" joint. (*B*) Lateral weight-bearing radiographs of feet with the different stages. Stage 1: minimal changes but positive Tc scan, with arrow pointing to a brightened area, including Harris lines; stages 2 to 4: progressive deformity with arrow indicating talar inclination axis; stage 5: complete extrusion of the navicular bone and marked equinization of the hindfoot. (*From* Maceira E. Aspectos clínicos y biomecánicos de la enfermedad de Müller-Weiss. Revista de Medicina y Cirugía del Pie 1996;10(1):58; with permission.)

patients with MWD.[21] Histologic samples through bone biopsy usually reveal no signs of osteonecrosis except in isolated bone fragments of the diseased navicular.[9]

MANAGEMENT OF MÜLLER-WEISS DISEASE

There is no gold standard treatment of patients with MWD. Various conservative and surgical interventions have been studied and reported to cause relief from mechanical

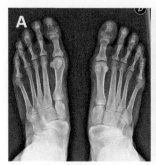 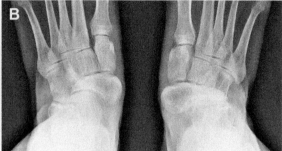

Fig. 8. Dorsoplantar weight-bearing radiograph showing (*A*) bilateral dysplasia of the navicular with index minus and (*B*) reduction of the talocalcaneal divergence with the talar head located over the anterior process of the calcaneus. Those references indicate subtalar varus deformity.

perinavicular pain.[22,23] Nonsurgical treatments should always be attempted first for MWD because they do not compromise future surgical treatment.

Conservative

Conservative treatment involves medications, offloading painful joints, padding, orthoses, adapted shoe wear modification, stretching exercises, and rocker-bottom shoes. There is no evidence to confirm the effectiveness of conservative measures for the treatment of MWD. However, most patients usually benefit from orthotic support if it is correctly indicated.

Rehabilitation
In the authors' experience magnetotherapy has been effective in temporally alleviating pain in around half of their MWD cases. However there is no published data on the efficacy of rehabilitation in MWD patients.

Shoe wear
Rocker-bottom shoes improve transition from the first to the third rocker and may alleviate perinavicular pain in some patients.[24]

Orthoses
Functional orthoses may be helpful to control abnormal hindfoot supination that definitely has an influence on pain in MWD. There are not many references to orthotic treatment of MWD.[10] In the authors' experience, most patients were referred to them with a diagnosis of perinavicular arthritis with valgus deformity. Insoles in these patients had medial arch support and a medial heel wedge to compensate for the apparent valgus deformity. Most patients were unsatisfied and complained of lateral ankle instability and peroneal pain when using the insoles. When the authors realized varus was a constant feature in their patients, they changed the type of orthotic design to fit the patients. A 10- to 12-mm lateral heel wedge helped to control subtalar supination, and medial arch support helped to reduce navicular sagging (**Fig. 9**). Conservative treatment with the use of rigid insoles with medial arch support and a lateral heel wedge to reduce supination of the heel has been effective in most of the authors' patients since then. Around 80% of their patients with *all* stages of MWD benefit from orthotic treatment and do not need surgery. Although it might be reasonable to think that patients who do not respond favorably to orthotics would also not respond favorably to surgery, the authors have observed no correlation between orthotic response and

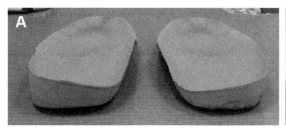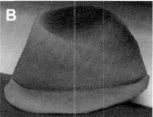

Fig. 9. Insoles for MWD with (*A*) lateral heel wedges to reduce supination of the heel and (*B*) medial arch support to reduce navicular sagging in the midfoot.

response to surgery. In fact, patients who showed no improvement with orthotics had considerable improvement following surgical treatment.

Those patients who fail to respond to insoles and experience severe pain and disability are candidates for surgery.

Surgical

In all patients who underwent surgical treatment, indications for surgery included the severity of pain and dysfunction rather than the stage of the disease or the response to orthotics. Different surgical procedures have been advocated for the treatment of MWD, including debridement of loose fragments, internal fixation of the navicular, and various types of arthrodesis (talonavicular, talonavicular-cuneiform, triple, and association of triple with naviculocuneiform fusion).[23,25]

Arthrodesis
Historically, surgical treatment of medial midfoot arthritis consisted of an arthrodesis of the affected joints (medial arch fusion or talonaviculocuneiform fusion). Watson-Jones[26] described fusion of the medial arch to treat sequelae of navicular fractures. The technique aims to restore the length of the medial column of the foot, which is desirable in a posttraumatic scenario but difficult to achieve in an MWD case.

Isolated talonavicular arthrodesis may be considered in the absence of naviculocuneiform arthritis, but it is associated with a high risk of nonunion.[27] Conventional fixation with screws may not be adequate to control adduction forces arising from the navicular nor lateral forces from the talus. The use of a lateral tension band in addition to medial screw fixation has been reported to be an effective alternative treatment to provide stability against deforming forces in MWD.[27] Fornaciari and colleagues[27] described the use of a lateral static tension band combined with 2 medial screws in 10 patients obtaining good radiological and clinical results with all patients being pain free at 2 years from surgery. Other investigators have also shown good results using isolated talonavicular fusion for MWD.[8,28]

Triple arthrodesis has been suggested for MWD patients when subtalar and calcaneocuboid joints were affected and in order to lower nonunion rates associated with isolated talonavicular fusion.[29] Open triple fusion has been reported to achieve bony union and improvement in a group of patients.[28] In situ arthroscopic triple arthrodesis has shown comparative results to the open procedure in all patients except one with persistent lateral foot pain after surgery.[30] Following a plantar pressure study in that patient, there was apparently a residual varus deformity suggesting that arthrodesis should ideally consider hindfoot varus correction in MWD.

Isolated talonavicular arthrodesis and triple arthrodesis do not address arthritis of the naviculocuneiform joint present in some MWD cases. When the naviculocuneiform joint is arthritic, *talonaviculocuneiform arthrodesis* has been considered by some groups to be the procedure of choice to restore medial arch and talocalcaneal alignment in MWD (**Fig. 10**).[31,32] Different techniques have been reported to achieve fusion with favorable reviews. Fernández de Retana and colleagues[16] used an autologous trapezoid graft through a dorsal approach to the medial column of the foot. A trapezoidal bed was carved along the dorsum of the talus to the cuneiform, and no fixation was used when the graft was stable. Cao and colleagues[31] performed a reverse V-shaped osteotomy through the talonavicular diseased joint and used a tricortical autogenous bone graft placed dorsally to achieve good clinical outcomes in 9 patients with MWD. Yu and colleagues[32] performed talonaviculocu neiform fusion in 7 MWD patients with a tricortical autologous iliac crest graft and fixation with plate and screws. Restoration of medial column length was noticed to be related to a good result.

Tan and colleagues[33] described the complete excision of the navicular and femoral head bone allograft interposition to fill the defect. The graft was fixed to the navicular and the cuneiform with an 8-hole low-contact plate achieving bone consolidation. Tosun and colleagues[34] reported on the removal of the fragmented bone and autologous bone grafting.

Osteotomies/joint-preserving surgery
Hindfoot arthrodesis procedures have many disadvantages, including the need for postoperative non-weight-bearing, a prolonged recovery time, a considerable rate of nonunion, the need for grafting, removal of metalwork, and loss of motion impacting alignment and adjacent joint function. Fusion techniques in MWD try to eliminate pain from arthritis, but pain is also caused by impaired biomechanics (hindfoot varus and medial arch deformity).

Some 15 years ago, when the authors recognized that hindfoot varus was responsible for most of the symptoms in MWD, they reviewed 15 of their patients that had undergone different types of fusions for MWD looking for factors influencing outcomes. Those cases in which hindfoot varus had been corrected properly had overall better outcomes with lower complication rates (including talonavicular nonunion).

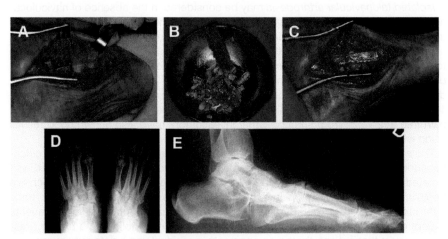

Fig. 10. Talonaviculocuneiform arthrodesis. (*A*) Preparation of joints and trapezoidal bed from talus to the cuneiform. (*B*) Preparation of autologous iliac crest bone graft. (*C*) Placing of tricortical graft along the bone bed. (*D*) Dorsoplantar and (*E*) lateral weight-bearing radiographs 1 year after surgery showing fusion and incorporation of the graft.

Talonavicular arthrodesis could not resolve joint incongruity in the naviculocuneiform joints, and fusion rates are known to be poor. In the authors' hands, it was not always easy to correct hindfoot varus at the time of fusion, and they found the need to use autologous bone grafting in some cases.

At around the same time, the authors observed that most of their MWD patients improved with lateral heel wedge and medial arch support insoles. Therefore, there had to be some degree of motion left in the perinavicular joint complex to allow for the orthotic support to shift the talus medially over the calcaneus and to change compressive forces from the diseased cartilage on the lateral navicular to the healthier cartilage on the medial navicular. Given the improvement most patients experienced with orthotic support, the authors went one step further by believing an isolated lateral sliding calcaneal osteotomy could improve symptoms in MWD patients.

From 2006 to 2016, the authors performed isolated calcaneal osteotomies, instead of fusions, on 18 patients with MWD. The osteotomy combined a conventional Dwyer lateral closing wedge osteotomy (around 8 mm) with lateral displacement calcaneal osteotomy (around 5–6 mm, reverse Koutsogiannis effect) (**Fig. 11**). Two 6.5-mm cannulated screws were used for fixation (**Fig. 12**). Weight-bearing was allowed at 3 weeks with the use of a walker boot and crutches. The authors explained to their patients during the informed consent process that calcaneal osteotomy may not always be successful and an arthrodesis might be necessary in the future. One patient has recently needed a secondary talonaviculocuneiform arthrodesis after not responding well enough to calcaneal osteotomy performed 4 years before. In this patient, there was a realignment of the talus following calcaneal osteotomy that made fusion much easier to be performed.

With an average follow-up of 4.5 years, 17 of the 18 noted improvement from the surgery, with American Orthopedic Foot and Ankle Society (AOFAS) foot function increased by 48 points and pain relief by 6 points on Visual Analogue Scale (VAS). Most of the patients are still doing well, with subjective rate of excellent results in 6 feet, good in 9 feet, and fair in 2 feet. No major complications were recorded. No differences were noticed with regard to staging and outcome. Radiographic changes were evident in all patients regardless of the initial images (**Fig. 13**). Improvement of the joint space was possibly due to the medial shifting of the navicular. Radiographic changes were present early in the postoperative period, and these changes ran parallel to clinical improvement in the authors' patients (**Fig. 14**). No patient showed

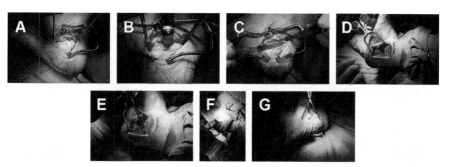

Fig. 11. Surgical technique for Dwyer osteotomy with lateral displacement. (*A*) Preparation of the lateral wall of the calcaneus via lateral approach. (*B*) Parallel cuts for Dwyer osteotomy. (*C*) Lateral wedge removed. (*D*) Lateral displacement of the posterior tuberosity of the calcaneus. (*E*) Removal of cancellous bone under the edge of the osteotomy. (*F*) Crushing of the lateral edge of the calcaneal tuberosity. (*G*) Closing the osteotomy before screw fixation.

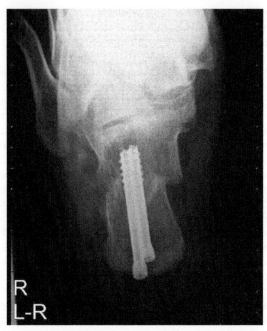

Fig. 12. Axial radiograph view showing the lateral displacement of the posterior tuberosity of the calcaneus. Cannulated headless 6.5-mm screws were used for fixation.

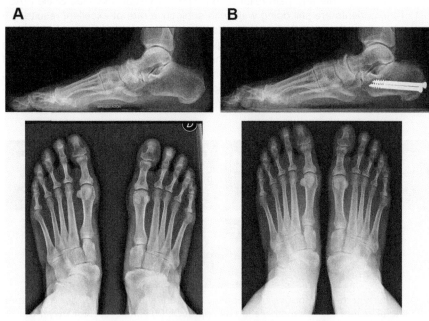

Fig. 13. Dorsoplantar and lateral weight-bearing radiograph (*A*) preoperatively and (*B*) 4 years postoperatively. The right talar head has shifted from lateral to medial following calcaneal osteotomy. Postoperative changes are especially evident at the talonavicular joint.

A   **B**

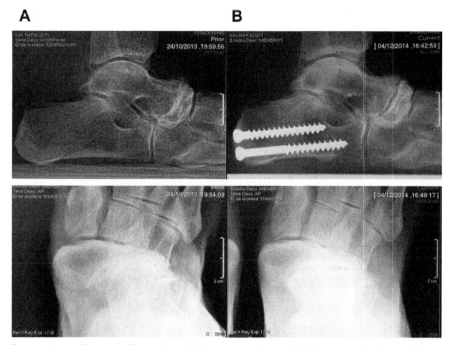

Fig. 14. Dorsoplantar and lateral weight-bearing radiograph (*A*) preoperatively and (*B*) just 6 months postoperatively.

worsening of the arthritis. One patient has undergone triple fusion 4 years from the index osteotomy surgery due to persistent perinavicular pain. Patients with no positive response to orthotics support posting the heel in valgus also benefited from calcaneal osteotomy (unpublished data).

In the authors' experience, patients with no improvement from orthotic support are also eligible for calcaneal osteotomy instead of fusion as the first indication for surgery. Although patients with advanced stages (3 and 4) of MWD might be candidates for fusion, most of the authors' patients at stages 3 to 5 responded well to the osteotomy. Calcaneal osteotomy has become the authors' procedure of choice regardless of the radiographic stage of the disease.

The authors' initial experience was shared with that of Myerson's group in Baltimore, Maryland, and results were comparable in terms of radiographic changes and clinical outcomes.[35] Dwyer calcaneal osteotomy combined with lateral displacement is a satisfactory treatment for the management of patients with MWD that had failed to respond to conservative measures. The follow-up is still relatively short, and the authors have reviewed a small number of cases, so they cannot predict how many of their patients will need an arthrodesis in the future. Calcaneal osteotomy has become their initial surgical procedure of choice in the treatment of MWD.

REFERENCES

1. Müller W. On an odd double-sided change of the tarsal navicular. Deutsche Zeitschrift für Chirurgie Leipzig 1927;201:84–7 [in German].
2. Weiss K. On the malacia of the tarsal navicular. Fortschritte auf dem Gebiete der Röntgenstrahlen 1927;45:63–7 [in German].

3. Müller W. On a typical deformity of the tarsal navicular and its clinical presentation. Fortschritte auf dem Gebiete der Röntgenstrahlen 1928;37:38–42 [in German].

4. Frosch L. The pathologic fracture of the tarsal navicular. Deutsche Zeitschrift für Chirurgie Leizpig 1931;232:487–92 [in German].

5. Volk C. Two cases of bipartite navicular. Z Orthop Ihre Grenzgeb 1937;66: 396–403 [in German].

6. Zimmer EA. Diseases, injuries and varieties of the tarsal navicular. Arch Orthop Trauma Surg 1937;38:396–411 [in German].

7. de Fine Licht E. On bipartite os naviculare pedis. Acta Radiol 1941;22:377–82.

8. Reade B, Atlas G, Distazio J, et al. Mueller-Weiss syndrome: an uncommon cause of midfoot pain. J Foot Ankle Surg 1998;37(6):535–9.

9. Maceira E. Clinical and biomechanical aspects of Müller Weiss disease. Revista de Medicina y Cirugía Del Pie 1996;10:53–65 [in Spanish].

10. Maceira E, Rochera R. Müller-Weiss disease: clinical and biomechanical features. Foot Ankle Clin 2004;9(1):105–25.

11. Simons B. Uber osteopathia deformans des os naviculare pedis. Z Orthop Chir 1930;52:564–8 [in German].

12. Brailsford JF. Osteochondritis of the adult tarsal navicular. J Bone Joint Surg Am 1939;26(1):111–20.

13. Fontaine R, Warter P, de Lange CH. The adult tarsal scaphoiditis (Müller-Weiss disease). J Radiol Electrol Med Nucl 1948;29:540–1 [in French].

14. Chambers CH. Congenital anomalies of the tarsal navicular with particular reference to calcaneo-navicular coalition. Br J Radiol 1950;23(274):580–6.

15. Kidner FC, Muro F. Köhler's disease of the tarsal scaphoid or os naviculare pedis retardatum. JAMA 1924;83(21):1650–4.

16. Fernández de Retana P, Maceira E, Fernández-Valencia JA, et al. Arthrodesis of the talonavicular-cuneiform joints in Müller-Weiss disease. Foot Ankle Clin 2004; 9(1):65–72.

17. Samim M, Moukaddam HA, Smitaman E. Imaging of Mueller-Weiss syndrome: a review of clinical presentations and imaging spectrum. Am J Roentgenol 2016; 207(2):W8–18.

18. Bartolotta R, McCullion J, Belfi L, et al. Mueller-Weiss syndrome: imaging and implications. Clin Imaging 2014;38:895–8.

19. Haller J, Sartoris DJ, Resnick D, et al. Spontaneous osteonecrosis of the tarsal navicular in adults: imaging findings. Am J Roentgenol 1998;151(2):355–8.

20. Welck MJ, Kaplan J, Myerson MS. Müller-Weiss syndrome: radiological features and the role of weightbearing computed tomography scan. Foot Ankle Spec 2016;9(3):245–51.

21. Hetsroni I, Nyska M, Ayalon M. Plantar pressure distribution in Patients with Müller-Weiss disease. Foot Ankle Int 2007;28(2):237–41.

22. Viladot A, Rochera R, Viladot A Jr. Necrosis of the navicular bone. Bull Hosp Jt Dis Orthop Inst 1987;47(2):285–93.

23. Mohiuddin T, Jennison T, Damany D. Müller-Weiss disease. Review of the current knowledge. Foot Ankle Surg 2014;20(2):79–84.

24. Myers KA, Long JT, Klein JP, et al. Biomechanical implications of the negative heel rocker sole shoe: gait kinematics and kinetics. Gait Posture 2006;24(3): 323–30.

25. Doyle T, Napier RJ, Wong-Chung J. Recognition and management of Müller-Weiss disease. Foot Ankle Int 2012;33(4):275–81.

26. Watson-Jones R. Fractures of the tarsal navicular bone. In: Watson-Jones R, editor. Fractures and joint injuries, vol. 2, 4th edition. Edinburgh (Scotland): E & S Livingstone; 1955. p. 900.

27. Fornaciari P, Gilgen A, Zwicky L, et al. Isolated talonavicular fusion with tension band for Müller-Weiss syndrome. Foot Ankle Int 2014;35(12):1316–22.

28. Wang X, Ma X, Zang C, et al. Flatfoot in Müller-Weiss syndrome: a case series. J Med Case Rep 2012;6:228.

29. Cao HH, Tang KL, Xu JZ. Peri-navicular arthrodesis for the stage III Müller-Weiss disease. Foot Ankle Int 2012;33(6):475–8.

30. Lui TH. Arthroscopic triple arthrodesis in patients with Müller Weiss disease. Foot Ankle Surg 2009;15(3):119–22.

31. Cao HH, Lu WZ, Tang KL. Isolated talonavicular arthrodesis and talonavicular-cuneiform arthrodesis for the Müller-Weiss disease. J Orthop Surg Res 2017; 12:83.

32. Yu G, Zhao Y, Zhou J, et al. Fusion of talonavicular and naviculocuneiform joints for the treatment of Müller-Weiss disease. J Foot Ankle Surg 2012;51(4):415–9.

33. Tan A, Smulders YC, Zöphel OT. Use of remodeled femoral head allograft for tarsal reconstruction in the treatment of Müller-Weiss disease. J Foot Ankle Surg 2011;50(6):721–6.

34. Tosun B, Al F, Tosun A. Spontaneous osteonecrosis of the tarsal navicular in an adult: Mueller-Weiss syndrome. J Foot Ankle Surg 2011;50(2):221–4.

35. Li S, Myerson M, Monteagudo M, et al. Efficacy of calcaneus osteotomy for treatment of symptomatic müller-weiss disease. Foot Ankle Int 2016;38(3):261–9.

Core Decompression and Bone Grafting for Osteonecrosis of the Talus: A Critical Analysis of the Current Evidence

Assem A. Sultan, MD[a], Michael A. Mont, MD[a,b],*

KEYWORDS

- Osteonecrosis • Talus • Core decompression • Bone grafting

KEY POINTS

- Core decompression is a relatively easy procedure from a technical standpoint and the results demonstrated it can be used with success to treat patients with early stage osteonecrosis of the talus.
- Percutaneous technique has also shown success and can be particularly useful in patients with polyarticular involvement who may have to undergo more invasive procedures for osteonecrosis of the hip, the knee, or other joints.
- Data on bone grafting are lacking, but it has been used mainly to treat traumatic patients who may benefit from augmenting the bony stalk.
- Vascularized grafts were the most commonly reported techniques in the literature but, because of their technical difficulty, it may not reflect a true estimate of their use and actual performance.
- Larger, prospective, multicenter studies are needed to guide specific patient selection criteria for each surgical intervention option.

Disclosure statement: Dr M.A. Mont is a consultant for, or has received institutional or research support from, the following companies: 3M, RefleXion Medical, PeerWell, Inc., age Products LLC, TissueGene, Inc., OnGoing Care Solutions Inc., DJO Global, MicroPort Orthopedics, Inc., OrthoSensor, Inc., National Institutes of Health, Stryker, Johnson & Johnson, Pacira Pharmaceuticals, Inc., and US Medical Innovations. Dr M.A. Mont is on the editorial/governing board of the *American Journal of Orthopedics*, the *Journal of Arthroplasty*, the *Journal of Knee Surgery*, and *Surgical Technology International*. He is a board or committee member of the American Academy of Orthopaedic Surgeons (AAOS). Dr A.A. Sultan has nothing to disclose.

[a] Department of Orthopaedic Surgery, Cleveland Clinic, 9500 Euclid Avenue, Cleveland, OH 44195, USA; [b] Strategic Initiatives, Lenox Hill Hospital, 100 E 77th Street, New York, NY 10075, USA
* Corresponding author. Department of Orthopaedic Surgery, Lenox Hill Hospital, New York, NY.
E-mail addresses: montm@ccf.org; rhondamont@aol.com

INTRODUCTION

Although less frequently encountered in clinical practice, osteonecrosis of the talus can have a devastating clinical sequalae leading to end-stage ankle joint destruction and loss of mobility, similar to hip and knee osteonecrosis.[1–3] Variability in etiology and presentation can contribute to a diagnostic challenge. Talar osteonecrosis is a common complication talar neck fractures.[3] Atraumatic cases are associated with chronic corticosteroid use, alcoholism, hyperuricemia, coagulopathies, or human immunodeficiency virus infection.[3–6] In atraumatic cases, patients typically present with polyarticular disease, posing an additional clinical challenge in the management. In addition, patients with atraumatic osteonecrosis may not have any identifiable risk factors[7] and may present with isolated osteonecrosis of the talus.[6]

Several operative treatments have been explored to treat patients with progressive or symptomatic disease that aim to alleviate pain and restore mobility. Because most of the affected patients are typically younger and more active individuals, joint preservation techniques have received increasing attention in this patient population. Core decompression, either through an open or percutaneous drilling approach, has been described. Similarly, nonvascularized and vascularized bone grafts have been used in clinical practice with varying results. In more advanced disease or when joint-preserving procedures fail, tibiotalar, talocalcaneal, triple arthrodesis, talectomy, or joint arthroplasty may be indicated.[2,8,9]

Owing to the relative paucity of studies, there is currently neither consensus nor clear guidelines for the optimal operative technique for various stages of talar osteonecrosis. In this review, we aimed to describe the surgical technique, and current evidence supporting the use of (1) core decompression and (2) bone grafting for treating osteonecrosis of the talus.

SURGICAL INDICATIONS

Core decompression and bone grafting techniques traditionally represent the first line of surgical treatment for symptomatic osteonecrosis of the talus following failure of nonsurgical management options. Core decompression has been performed mainly in Ficat stage I and II talar osteonecrosis to relieve pain and improve the function and are not suitable when the talas has collapsed lesions. The indications are less clear for bone grafting and current evidence regarding these techniques comes from small case series that was performed mainly in posttraumatic osteonecrosis. In studies that reported the utilization of bone grafting techniques, patients mainly had Ficat stage II and III osteonecrosis. Therefore, it represent a salvage procedure for precollapse stages and may help to avoid the need for ankle arthrodesis or arthroplasty. It is important to note that an experienced surgeon with prior familiarity with the techniques for bone grafting is another specific prerequisite for this option to be considered when indicated.

SURGICAL TECHNIQUE
Core Decompression

This technique can be performed either through a conventional or a minimally invasive approach. In the conventional core decompression, a standard anterolateral or anteromedial approach to the talar dome is used to insert a trocar under fluoroscopic guidance to access the area of osteonecrosis visualized in preoperative imaging studies. Biopsy can be obtained and drilling can then be carried out. Multiple passes can be made as necessary, taking care not to injure the articular cartilage. Modification of the conventional technique into minimally invasive have been described by Marulanda and colleagues. They reported inserting a 3.2-mm percutaneous Steinman pin starting beneath the medial malleolus under fluoroscopic guidance. The pin can be passed to the exact location of the lesion and a core can be removed for the desired location.

Bone grafting

In all studies that reported on bone grafting methods, only vascularized harvesting techniques were used. Yu and colleagues[10] reported using a transposed vascularized cuneiform bone flap accompanied by local augmentation with iliac cancellous bone graft. Zhang and colleagues[11] reported harvesting vascularized grafts from the first cuneiform bone with the malleolaris anteriomedialis or the medial tarsal arteries in 13 patients. In addition, they also used vascularized cuboid bone graft with the lateral tarsal artery in 11 patients. Doi and Sakai[12] used vascularized corticoperiosteal bone graft nourished by the articular branch of the descending genicular artery and vein from the supracondylar region of the femur. More recently, Nunley and Hamid[13] reported on the results of vascularized pedicle bone grafting technique form the cuboid. The tibiotalar joint is accessed anteriorly and a guide pin in inserted under fluoroscopic guidance to the specific lesion in correlation with the preoperative imaging. A series of sequential drillings, curettage, and burring is used to debride the lesion and create a tunnel through which the harvested graft can be implanted. The graft is obtained from a territory of the cuboid bone consistently supplied by the proximal lateral tarsal artery. The tourniquet is removed and the graft is checked for perfusion after harvesting and before implantation. For all bone grafting techniques, strict non–weight-bearing is advised for up to 3 months after surgery to allow for undisturbed healing of the graft.

TREATMENT OUTCOMES
Surgical Results

Core decompression

A total of 4 studies have investigated core decompression and its outcomes in 199 ankles and 139 patients all had atraumatic osteonecrosis of the talus. There were 96 women and 43 men. All 4 studies were retrospective case series studies (Level IV). Mean weighted follow-up time in these studies was 5.6 years (range, 2–15 years).

Patients who underwent core decompression had grade I or II osteonecrosis of the talus in 2 studies,[6,14,15] whereas Delanois and colleagues[16] also included patients who had grades III and IV osteonecrosis (9 of 37 ankles). All studies used the Ficat and Arlet system[17] modified for the ankle.[14] In all studies, patient had atraumatic etiologies and the most common identified risk factor was chronic corticosteroid use (>5 mg/d) ranging between 52% and 83% of patients. In 2 studies,[15,16] most patients had polyarticular involvement of osteonecrosis reaching up to 58% of patients in the study by Marulanda and colleagues[15] and 63% in the study by Delanois and colleagues. In 1 study, 32% of patients had a previous drilling attempt and Delanois and colleagues[16] reported that the mean time from diagnosis to surgery averaged 5 months in their cohort. In all studies, patient underwent partial weight-bearing (up to 50%) for 4 to 6 weeks postoperatively then advanced to full weight-bearing based on clinical and radiographic follow-up progress.

Mont and colleagues[14] and Delanois and colleagues[16] reported clinical outcomes using the Mazur ankle grading system. Pooled results from these studies showed improvement in clinical outcomes from a score of 34 points preoperatively to 90 points postoperatively. In the study by Marulanda and colleagues,[15] patients also exhibited clinical improvement using the American Orthopaedic Foot and Ankle Society–Hindfoot and Ankle (AOFAS-HFA) score, from 42 points preoperatively to 88 points postoperatively. In the study by Issa and colleagues,[6] 83% of patients did not have further disease progression clinically or radiologically. Clinical outcomes were evaluated using the AOFAS-HFA score, the University of California Los Angeles activity score, visual analog scale for pain, and Short-Form 36 scores (SF-36). The authors reported a significant improvement in the mean AOFAS-HFA (P = .001), the mean University of California Los Angeles activity scores (P = .025), and the mean visual analog scale pain scores (P = .001). The mean final SF-36 physical component score was 44 points (range, 21–65 points) and the mean final SF-36 mental component score was 52.5 points (range, 29–68 points). Among all studies, approximately 21% of patients progressed from stage I to II or stage II to III at mean follow-up of 5.6 years (range, 2–15 years).[6,15,16] Additionally, 11% of patients required ankle fusion.[14–16]

Bone grafting

A total of 5 studies have investigated the use of bone grafting techniques and its outcomes in 64 patients, of which, 22 had atraumatic osteonecrosis, 5 had posttraumatic osteonecrosis, and in 37 patients, no specific etiology was reported.[10–12,18] All 5 studies were retrospective case series studies (Level IV). The mean follow-up time was extrapolated from 3 studies and ranged between 14 months and 2 years. Only Yu and colleagues[10] reported on the preoperative Ficat grade for their cohort, with 8 at stage II, 10 at stage III, and 3 at stage IV.

Outcomes Yu and colleagues[10] reported their clinical outcomes using the Kenwright criteria which were excellent in 8, good in 10, fair in 1, and poor in 1 patient. Radiologically the necrotic area was filled with newly formed bone with a reported excellent to good rate of 90% filling. Zhang and colleagues reported that 16 of 24 patients had normal or near normal function of the ankle joint between 3.0 and 5.5 years at final follow-up with excellent radiological outcomes. Doi and colleagues[12,18] used pain scores and the presence of collapse to report their outcomes with 6 of 7 patients having no pain or collapse at final follow-up. Nunley and Hamid[13] reported on vascularized cuboid grafting technique in 13 patients with mean follow-up of 6 years (range, 2–12 years). In total, 2 patients failed and required total ankle arthroplasty. For the remaining patients, they demonstrated clinical improvement as measured by 23.3 ± 18.9 points and 39.4 ± 10.1 points improvement postoperatively in SF-36 physical and mental components questionnaires, respectively.

SUMMARY

Compared with osteonecrosis of the hip or knee, data are lacking on the natural history, detailed risk factors, and ideal treatment for osteonecrosis of the talus. Atraumatic cases have been mainly linked to chronic corticosteroid use as the most commonly identified risk factor. Current evidence suggest that core decompression can be performed with successful outcome particularly in patients with early and traumatic disease (stages I and II). Bone grafting has been mainly used in patients with traumatic osteonecrosis and less commonly used to treat patients with atraumatic osteonecrosis. Vascularized bone grafting was the main technique reported in the literature. However, these procedures are typically challenging to perform from a technical standpoint and may not be available for every patient when indicated.

This review is not without limitations. Our analysis is based on the quality of the published literature, most of which were of low-level evidence of retrospective case series. Additionally, current studies reported outcomes with a mean follow-up of 5 years, which may not reflect the true performance of the investigated procedures.

Nevertheless, in this review we adopted a comprehensive approach, encompassing all published studies on core decompression or bone grating for talar osteonecrosis.

The surgical technique for core decompression is relatively easier and carries less morbidity to the patient compared with bone grafting. The technique first described by Mont and colleagues[14] using a standard anteromedial and anterolateral open approaches to the talus. A large diameter trocar is used to remove a cylinder of bone under fluoroscopic visualization. Preoperative MRI evaluation aids in deciding the area of the talus to be cannulated. A minimally invasive percutaneous technique was developed and reported by Marulanda and colleagues[15] and Mont and colleagues[14] using a 3.2 Steinman pin under fluoroscopy by starting beneath the medial malleolus and penetrating the talus. The pin is then advanced to the desired area where the bulk of osteonecrotic lesion is. The authors suggested this technique may be associated with less incidence of articular cartilage damage and respects the anatomic considerations for the small sized talus. Surgery can also be done on outpatient basis.[6]

Studies that reported on bone grafting mainly included patients who had traumatic osteonecrosis. Vascularized bone graft can be harvested from the first cuneiform, cuboid, or supracondylar region of the femur. The latter technique was described by Doi and colleagues,[12,18] in the which the descending genicular vessels are mobilized from their origin from the adductor magnus to their termination over the periosteum of the medial condylar and supracondylar areas of the femur. A sharp chisel is then used to harvest a full-thickness corticocancellous graft taking care to keep the overlaying periosteum intact and transposed to the talus. To the best of author's knowledge the nonvascularized technique has been described mainly in previous case reports using iliac crest bone graft.[3]

In conclusion, core decompression is a relatively easy procedure from a technical standpoint and the results demonstrated it can be used with success to treat patients with early stage osteonecrosis of the talus. Percutaneous technique has also shown success and can be particularly useful in patients with polyarticular involvement who may have to undergo more invasive procedures for osteonecrosis of the hip, the knee, or other joints. Data on bone grafting is lacking but it has been used mainly to treat traumatic patients who may benefit from augmenting the bony stalk. Vascularized grafts were the most commonly reported technique in the literature but because of their technical difficulty, it may not reflect a true estimate of their use and actual performance. Larger, prospective, multicenter studies are needed to guide the specific patient selection criteria for each surgical intervention option.

REFERENCES

1. Mont MA, Jones LC, Hungerford DS. Nontraumatic osteonecrosis of the femoral head: ten years later. J Bone Joint Surg Am 2006;88(5):1117–32.
2. Manes HR, Alvarez E, Llevine LS. Preliminary report of total ankle arthroplasty for osteonecrosis of the talus. Clin Orthop Relat Res 1977;127:200–2.
3. Horst F, Gilbert BJ, Nunley JA. Avascular necrosis of the talus: current treatment options. Foot Ankle Clin 2004;9(4):757–73.
4. Gayton JC, Burleson D, Polenakovik H, et al. Avascular necrosis of the talus in a HIV-infected patient. Foot Ankle Int 2010;31(12):1111–4.
5. Orth P, Anagnostakos K. Coagulation abnormalities in osteonecrosis and bone marrow edema syndrome. Orthopedics 2013;36(4):290–300.
6. Issa K, Naziri Q, Kapadia BH, et al. Clinical characteristics of early-stage osteonecrosis of the ankle and treatment outcomes. J Bone Joint Surg Am 2014;96(9): e73.

7. Dall D, Macnab I. Spontaneous avascular necrosis of the talus: a report of two cases. S Afr Med J 1970;44(7):193–6.

8. Devries JG, Philbin TM, Hyer CF. Retrograde intramedullary nail arthrodesis for avascular necrosis of the talus. Foot Ankle Int 2010;31(11):965–72.

9. Haverstock BD, Barth LD, Jacobs AM. Ankle arthrodesis following avascular necrosis of the talus in a patient with lupus. J Am Podiatr Med Assoc 1997;87(10): 483–9.

10. Yu X, Zhao D, Sun Q, et al. Treatment of non-traumatic avascular talar necrosis by transposition of vascularized cuneiform bone flap plus iliac cancellous bone grafting. Zhonghua Yi Xue Za Zhi 2010;90(15):1035–8 [in Chinese].

11. Zhang Y, Liu Y, Jiang Y. Treatment of avascular necrosis of talus with vascularized bone graft. Zhongguo Xiu Fu Chong Jian Wai Ke Za Zhi 1998;12(5):285–7 [in Chinese].

12. Doi K, Sakai K. Vascularized periosteal bone graft from the supracondylar region of the femur. Microsurgery 1994;15(5):305–15.

13. Nunley JA, Hamid KS. Vascularized pedicle bone-grafting from the cuboid for talar osteonecrosis. J Bone Jt Surg 2017;99(10):848–54.

14. Mont MA, Schon LC, Hungerford MW, et al. Avascular necrosis of the talus treated by core decompression. J Bone Joint Surg Br 1996;78(5):827–30.

15. Marulanda GA, McGrath MS, Ulrich SD, et al. Percutaneous drilling for the treatment of atraumatic osteonecrosis of the ankle. J Foot Ankle Surg 2010;49(1): 20–4.

16. Delanois RE, Mont MA, Yoon TR, et al. Atraumatic osteonecrosis of the talus. J Bone Joint Surg Am 1998;80(4):529–36.

17. Ficat RP. Aseptic necrosis of the femur head. Pathogenesis: the theory of circulation. Acta Orthop Belg 1981;47(2):198–9 [in French].

18. Doi K, Hattori Y. Vascularized bone graft from the supracondylar region of the femur. Microsurgery 2009;29(5):379–84.

Avascular Necrosis of the Tibial Plafond Following Rotational Ankle Fractures

Angela K. Heinen, DO[a],*, Thomas G. Harris, MD[a,b]

KEYWORDS

- Osteonecrosis • Tibia • Plafond • Ankle • Fracture

KEY POINTS

- Avascular necrosis following rotational ankle fractures is most commonly described in the talus; however, it can also occur in the tibial plafond. These sequelae of ankle fractures are rarely described in the literature.
- Avascular necrosis of the distal tibia after rotational ankle fractures must be included in the differential diagnosis in patients who continue to have pain despite radiographic healing of the fractures.
- Diagnosis of avascular necrosis of the distal tibia is best confirmed with MRI of the involved extremity.
- Treatment options for this condition include observation, limited weight-bearing, bisphosphonates, hyperbaric oxygen therapy, shock wave therapy, pulsed wave electromagnetic field therapy and physical therapy, and surgical options such as percutaneous drilling, debridement with bone grafting (vascularized and nonvascularized), arthrodesis, and total ankle arthroplasty.

INTRODUCTION

Avascular necrosis (AVN) is described as the cellular death within bone caused by a lack of circulation (**Fig. 1**).[1] Several pathogenic mechanisms may result in ischemia and AVN, including vascular interruption, intravascular occlusion, and intraosseous extravascular compression.[2] Issa and colleagues[3] examined the clinical characteristics of early stage osteonecrosis of the ankle and found the most common identifiable risk factors for nontraumatic osteonecrosis to be chronic corticosteroid use, alcohol abuse, tobacco use, hypertension, and systemic lupus erythematosus. Trauma remains the most common mechanical cause of osteonecrosis throughout the body, particularly in the ankle.[4] **Box 1** references common conditions associated with osteonecrosis.

Disclosures: The authors have nothing to disclose.
[a] Foot and Ankle Surgery, UCLA Harbor Medical Center, 1000 W. Carson Street, Torrance, CA 90502, USA; [b] Foot and Ankle Department, Congress Medical Associates, 800 South Raymond, 2nd Floor, Pasadena, CA 91105, USA
* Corresponding author. 800 South Raymond, 2nd Floor, Pasadena, CA 91105.
E-mail address: drheinen34@gmail.com

Foot Ankle Clin N Am 24 (2019) 113–119
https://doi.org/10.1016/j.fcl.2018.10.003
1083-7515/19/© 2018 Elsevier Inc. All rights reserved.

foot.theclinics.com

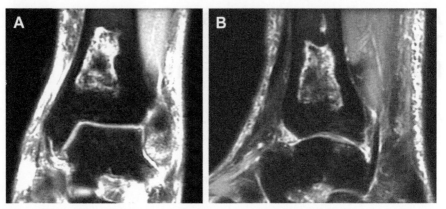

Fig. 1. Coronal (*A*) and sagittal (*B*) MRI views show an area of AVN of the tibial plafond.

AVN of the ankle following trauma most commonly occurs and is best described in the talus. AVN of the distal tibial plafond following ankle fractures is a known complication as well but has rarely been described in the literature. Assal and colleagues[5] published a case series of 9 patients who developed osteonecrosis of the lateral tibial plafond following ankle fractures. Another retrospective case series by Blanke and colleagues[6] examined the rates of osteonecrosis in 28 patients following open fracture

---

Box 1
Common conditions associated with osteonecrosis

Mechanical
  Trauma

Hematologic
  Sickle cell anemia
  Hemophilia

Metabolic
  Gaucher's disease
  Diabetes
  Gout
  Pancreatitis

Rheumatologic
  Systemic lupus erythematosus
  Rheumatoid arthritis

Infectious diseases
  Osteomyelitis
  HIV infection

Iatrogenic
  Corticosteroids
  Alcoholism
  Cigarette smoking
  Dysbaric osteonecrosis (The bends)
  Bisphosphonate use
  Radiation therapy

Abbreviation: HIV, human immunodeficiency virus.

dislocations of the ankle. To the authors' knowledge, beyond these 2 case series, there have been 2 other adult[7,8] and 6 pediatric cases described.[9–13]

DIAGNOSIS

Following ankle fractures, it is routine practice to obtain serial radiographs to assess for radiographic healing of the fractures. The development of AVN of the tibial plafond must be included in the differential diagnosis if the patient continues to have pain despite evidence of radiographic healing. In a case series by Assal and colleagues,[5] radiographs showed advanced signs of AVN of the lateral tibial plafond at a mean time of 5.9 months following injury. Patients with these sequelae of ankle fractures often have continued pain, swelling, and activity limitations despite evidence of radiographic healing of the fractures. Mechanical symptoms may also be present. One must be observant to clinical signs and symptoms of infection. This can be ruled out by obtaining inflammatory markers (erythrocyte sedimentation rate, C-reactive protein, leukocytes) and a joint aspirate if warranted, to diagnose or rule out infection.

If infection has been ruled out, one must further investigate the possibility of AVN. Radiographs are limited in their use of diagnosing AVN. Conventional radiographs are useful for the diagnosis only after the development of sclerosis, articular collapse, or a crescent sign.[1] Other diagnostic imaging studies can be considered, including a nuclear bone scan, single-photon emission computed tomography, or PET scanning. However, the gold standard for diagnosing AVN, once infection or other causes of pain have been ruled out, remains MRI.

MRI findings in the setting of osteonecrosis will include surrounding bone marrow edema and focal defects in the distal tibial articular surface. Diffuse marrow edema is seen in early osteonecrosis and produces a low signal intensity on T1-weighted images and a high signal intensity on T2-weighted images. In advanced stages of the disease, both T1-and T2-weighted images demonstrate low signal intensity.[4]

McLeod and colleagues[14] described a case of nontraumatic osteonecrosis of the distal tibia. Their patient had a history of ulcerative colitis and use of high-dose steroids in the acute stage of the condition. Although trauma is the most common cause, many other factors can be associated with osteonecrosis in not only the foot but throughout the body. These conditions associated with osteonecrosis can be referenced in **Table 1**. Staging for osteonecrosis was originally described by Ficat and this system references the femoral head.

Specifically, patients with pronation external rotation (PER) ankle fractures should be observed for the development of AVN of the lateral tibial plafond. Menck and colleagues[15] demonstrated that the lateral tibial epiphysis is relatively less vascularized than the medial part. In a study by Rajagopalan and colleagues,[8] they theorized that it is the susceptibility of the posterior ligamentous-capsular structures of the posterior ankle that predisposes the posterolateral tibial plafond to osteonecrosis. Their patient had a small avulsion off the posterior ankle, suggesting a posterior capsular injury. Surgeons should have a heightened awareness for the risk of developing AVN of the tibial plafond in these patients with PER ankle fractures and an avulsion fracture off the posterior tibia.

TREATMENT OPTIONS

There are many treatment options for distal tibial osteonecrosis. Much of the literature on the treatment of distal tibial AVN is based on the literature from the treatment of femoral head AVN. Nonoperative treatments of AVN in the talus include limited weight-bearing with or without bracing.[16] Conservative medical management is

Table 1	
Ficat femoral head osteonecrosis staging system	
Stage 0	Normal radiograph
	Normal MRI
	Asymptomatic patient
Stage 1	Normal radiograph
	Abnormal MRI
	Symptomatic patient
Stage 2	Abnormal radiograph with subchondral sclerosis or cystic changes
	MRI shows geographic edema
	Symptomatic patient with pain and stiffness
Stage 3	Abnormal radiograph with crescent sign visible
	MRI shows crescent sign
	Patient with pain, stiffness, and limp
Stage 4	Abnormal radiograph with degenerative changes of the acetabulum with decreased joint space
	MRI shows degenerative joint disease
	Patient with pain and limp

usually the first line of treatment but has historically yielded relatively poor results especially in cases with femoral head AVN.

MEDICAL TREATMENTS

Medical treatments including bisphosphonates have been shown to be effective in many animal models especially for femoral head AVN.[17] These medications are thought to be effective by reducing osteoclast activity, which can reduce bone edema and remodeling in affected areas. Therefore, they would increase bone mineral density and hence delay the progression of bony collapse. However, bisphosphonates have not been specifically studied for distal tibial AVN. Several studies have investigated the protective effects of the statins in reversing corticosteroid-related femoral head AVN. Pritchett[18] retrospectively reviewed data from 284 patients who had received high-dose steroids and were also taking a statin. They noted a 1% rate of AVN, which was a significantly lower rate compared with that in who were not on a statin (3%–20%). Again, statins have not been investigated specifically with respect to distal tibial AVN. Other nonoperative measures that have been described include hyperbaric oxygen therapy, shock wave therapy, pulsed wave electromagnetic field therapy, and physical therapy.[19]

SURGICAL TREATMENTS

Surgical options include percutaneous drilling, debridement with bone grafting (vascularized and nonvascularized), arthrodesis, and total ankle arthroplasty. The precise indications for these procedures continue to be controversial.[3] Further, the role of arthroscopy is yet to be determined based on the current literature for distal tibial osteonecrosis. Lastly, the timing of operative intervention is also controversial. Just as with the hip, initial surgical correction of distal tibial AVN is aimed at sparing the joint, especially in early stages of AVN without collapse. Marulanda and colleagues[20] studied the treatment of distal tibial AVN with a new technique using multiple (1–3) small percutaneous 3 mm perforations in a total of 44 ankles. At an average follow-up of 45 months, 40 ankles (91%) had achieved a successful clinical outcome and an improvement in their mean American Orthopedic Foot and Ankle Society score, which improved from 42 to 88. No complications were seen, but 3 ankles subsequently collapsed and required arthrodesis.

SURGICAL TECHNIQUES
Percutaneous Drilling

When performing percutaneous drilling of distal tibial AVN, it is important to pass the drill through vascularized bone into the avascular bone so as to encourage angiogenesis through the new channels. This type of technique differs slightly than the typical core decompression done in the femoral head in that the caliber of drills is much smaller and the goal of treatment is not removal of necrotic bone but rather angiogenesis. This is in part due to the smaller-sized bone encountered in the distal tibia versus proximal femur. It is thought to be less invasive and removes less bone than core decompression.[20]

The authors usually use a cannulated drill system when performing this type of surgery. The size of the lesion and the size of the patient will help determine what size of a drill to use. For a larger patient weighing more than 250 pounds a cannulated 3.0 mm drill bit is used with a 4.0 mm- or 4.5 mm-sized screw. For a smaller patient between 150 and 250 pounds, a 2.0 mm- or 2.5 mm-sized cannulated drill is used, as seen in **Fig. 2**B. The authors prefer to use multiple (2–4 total) passes into the lesion with a smaller drill from different areas and trajectories rather than a single pass with a larger-sized (5–6 mm) drill to help increase angiogenesis from different areas. The cannulated nature of the drill allows us to use a smaller-sized K-Wire first to make sure the wire is in the correct position in both anteroposterior and lateral radiographic planes before actually drilling, as seen in **Fig. 2**A. The authors do not typically back fill the channels created by the drilling with demineralized bone matrix.

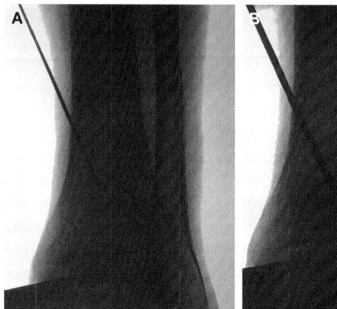
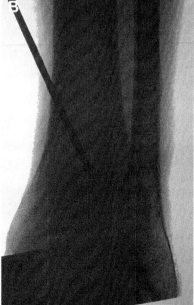

Fig. 2. Intraoperative radiographs show percutaneous localization of the area of AVN (*A*), followed by drilling of the defect with a cannulated drill (*B*).

Postoperatively, the patient is placed into a well-padded splint for 1 week and told to be non–weight-bearing. After 1 week, they are converted to a tall constrained ankle motion boot, and their weight-bearing is increased to partial weight-bearing of 25% to 50%. At this point, gentle active but non–weight-bearing range of motion exercises are instituted a few times a day. After 2 weeks, they are increased to weight-bearing as tolerated with the goal being to be full weight-bearing by 3 to 4 weeks postoperatively. The boot can usually be discontinued 4 to 6 weeks after the procedure. At this point, the authors still support the ankle with a lace up ankle brace until 12 weeks postoperatively.

Ankle Arthrodesis

In terms of ankle arthrodesis for distal tibial AVN, the method of arthrodesis depends on whether significant tibial collapse has occurred or not. If the patient has failed percutaneous drilling with respect to continued pain but no collapse, another attempt at percutaneous drilling or open bone grafting would be reasonable. However, if there is collapse of the distal tibial and a resultant deformity then arthrodesis is the best surgical option.

Total Ankle Arthroplasty

Total ankle arthroplasty should be approached with caution in this situation given the risk of future subsidence. If there is significant deformity (greater than 10–15° of coronal or sagittal plane malalignment), then an open arthrodesis with correction of the deformity should be undertaken.

SUMMARY

Osteonecrosis of the tibial plafond following rotational ankle fractures is a rarely described entity in the literature. This must be included in the differential diagnosis in patients who continue to have pain despite radiographic healing of the fractures. Diagnosis of AVN of the distal tibia is best confirmed with MRI of the involved extremity. Treatment options of this condition include observation, limited weight-bearing, bisphoshonates, hyperbaric oxygen therapy, shock wave therapy, pulsed wave electromagnetic field therapy and physical therapy, and surgical options such as percutaneous drilling, debridement with bone grafting (vascularized and nonvascularized), arthrodesis, and possibly total ankle arthroplasty.

FUTURE CONSIDERATIONS

Future research on this topic could include more anatomic or cadaver studies about specifically why AVN occurs in the lateral versus medial tibial plafond. Biological adjuvant treatments, such as juvenile allogeneic chondrocyte implantation (JACI; DeNovo NT Natural Tissue Graft; Zimmer, Warsaw, IN) with autologous bone marrow aspirate concentrate have been studied in the talus[21]; however, there have not been any studies performed specifically for these adjuvants in the tibial plafond. Subchondroplasty has been indicated in the treatment for bone marrow lesions in the foot and ankle as a joint sparing procedure. These techniques could be further studied for treatment of areas of AVN in the foot and ankle to determine its efficacy for these types of lesions. The overall use of orthobiologics has been scarcely studied in the foot and ankle realm. There should be further studies about their use in foot and ankle surgical treatment of AVN.

REFERENCES

1. DiGiovanni CW, Patel A, Calfee R, et al. Osteonecrosis in the foot. J Am Acad Orthop Surg 2007;15:208–17.

2. Shah KN, Racine J, Jones LC, et al. Pathophysiology and risk factors for osteo-necrosis. Curr Rev Musculoskelet Med 2015;8(3):201–9.
3. Issa K, Naziri Q, Kapadia B, et al. Clinical characteristics of early-stage osteonec-rosis of the ankle and treatment outcomes. J Bone Joint Surg Am 2014;96:e73.
4. Assouline-Dayan Y, Chang C, Greenspan A, et al. Pathogenesis and natural his-tory of osteonecrosis. Semis Arthritis Rheum 2002;32:94–124.
5. Assal M, Sangeorzan B, Hansen S. Post-traumatic osteonecrosis of the lateral tibial plafond. Foot Ankle Surg 2007;13:24–9.
6. Blanke F, Lowe S, Ferrat P, et al. Osteonecrosis of distal tibia in open dislocation fractures of the ankle. Injury 2014;45:1659–63.
7. Chakravarty D, Khanna A, Kumar A. Post-traumatic osteonecrosis of distal tibia. Injury Extra 2007;38:262–6.
8. Rajagopalan S, Lloyd J, Upadhyay V, et al. Osteonecrosis of the distal tibia after a pronation external rotation ankle fracture: literature review and management. J Foot Ankle Surg 2011;50:445–8.
9. Siffert R, Arlin A. Post-traumatic aseptic necrosis of the distal tibial epiphysis. J Bone Joint Surg Am 1950;32-A:691.
10. Robertson D. Post-traumatic osteochondritis of the lower tibial epiphysis. J Bone Joint Surg Am 1964;46:212–3.
11. Gasco J, Gonzalez-Herranz P, Minguez MF, et al. Avascular necrosis of distal tibial epiphysis: report of two cases. J Pediatr Orthop B 2010;19:361–5.
12. Pugely A, Nemeth B, McCarthy J, et al. Osteonecrosis of the distal tibia metaphy-sis after a salter-harris i injury: a case report. J Orthop Trauma 2012;26:e11–5.
13. Bhattacharjee A, Singh J, Mangham D, et al. Osteonecrosis of the distal tibial metaphysis after Salter-Harris type-2 injury: a case report. J Pediatr Orthop B 2015;24:366–9.
14. McLeod J, Ng A, Kruse D, et al. Nontraumatic osteonecrosis of the distal tibia: a case presentation and review of the literature. J Foot Ankle Surg 2017;56:158–66.
15. Menck J, Bertram C, Lierse W. Sectorial angioarchitecture of the human tibia. Acta Anat 1992;143(1):67–73.
16. Horst F, Gilbert B, Nunley J. Avascular necrosis of the talus: current treatment op-tions. Foot Ankle Clin N Am 2004;9(4):757–73.
17. Rajpura A, Wright A, Board T. Medical management of osteonecrosis of the hip: a review. Hip Int 2011;21(04):385–92.
18. Pritchett J. Statin therapy decreases the risk of osteonecrosis in patients receiving steroids. Clin Orthop Relat Res 2011;386:173–8.
19. Vulpiani M, Vetrano M, Trischitta D, et al. Extracorporeal shock wave therapy in early osteonecrosis of the femoral head: prospective clinical study with long-term follow-up. Arch Orthop Trauma Surg 2012;132(4):499–508.
20. Marulanda G, McGrath M, Ulrich S, et al. Percutaneous drilling for the treatment of atraumatic osteonecrosis of the ankle. J Foot Ankle Surg 2010;49(1):20–4.
21. DeSandis BA, Haleem AM, Sofka CM, et al. Arthroscopic treatment of osteochon-dral lesions of the talus using juvenile articular cartilage allograft and autologous bone marrow aspirate concentration. J Foot Ankle Surg 2018;57(2):273–80.

Vascularized Pedicle Graft for Talar Osteonecrosis

Elizabeth A. Cody, MD[a], James A. Nunley, MD[b],*

KEYWORDS

- Vascularized pedicle graft • Vascularized bone graft • Talar avascular necrosis

KEY POINTS

- Vascularized bone grafting for talar osteonecrosis is a good treatment option for patients with talar osteonecrosis in the absence of significant subchondral collapse and tibiotalar arthritis.
- Vascularized bone grafts may be harvested from the cuboid using the proximal lateral tarsal artery as a pedicle. Smaller grafts with less excursion may be harvested from the medial and lateral cuneiforms.
- Outcomes in small case series have been promising, with more than 80% of patients requiring no additional surgery.

INTRODUCTION

Osteonecrosis of the talus is a difficult clinical problem without reliable treatment options. It is staged using the Ficat and Arlet system, modified for the ankle (**Table 1**).[1,2] Nonoperative management of talar osteonecrosis has had limited success, with about one in three patients ultimately requiring surgical intervention.[3] Patients who have failed nonoperative management may be treated with surgical options encompassing joint-sparing and joint-sacrificing procedures.

Joint-sacrificing procedures can include talar replacement or arthrodesis. In cases where the extent of disease is limited, total ankle arthroplasty may also be a viable option. Joint-sacrificing procedures are generally used in more advanced osteonecrosis with joint collapse and arthritis (stage IV).

Joint-sparing procedures are reserved for earlier stage disease, in which subchondral collapse is absent or minimal. Core decompression[4–7] and vascularized bone grafting[8–10] can lead to improved vascularity and prevent or delay further degeneration

Disclosure Statement: The authors have nothing to disclose.
[a] Duke University Medical Center, 40 Duke Medicine Circle, Durham, NC 27710, USA;
[b] Department of Orthopaedic Surgery, Duke University Medical Center, 40 Duke Medicine Circle, Durham, NC 27710, USA
* Corresponding author.
E-mail address: james.nunley@duke.edu

Table 1 Ficat and Arlet staging of osteonecrosis (modified for the ankle)	
Stage	**Radiographic Findings**
I	Normal
II	Cystic and/or sclerotic lesions, normal talar contour, no subchondral fractures
III	Crescent sign, subchondral collapse
IV	Joint space narrowing, secondary tibial cysts, osteophytes, arthritic changes

Data from Arlet J, Ficat R. Forage-biopsie de la tête fémorale dans l'ostéonécrose primitive. Observations histo-pathologiques portent sur nuit forages. Rev Rhum 1964;31:257–64; and Gross CE, Sershon RA, Frank JM, et al. Treatment of osteonecrosis of the talus. JBJS Rev 2016;4(7):https://doi.org/10.2106/JBJS.RVW.15.00087.

in most patients. This article focuses on the indications, technique, and outcomes of vascularized pedicle grafts for talar osteonecrosis.

INDICATIONS

The primary indication for vascularized bone grafting is osteonecrosis with minimal subchondral collapse (stages II and III) and less than 60% talar involvement on MRI. Contraindications include greater than 1 mm of articular collapse and presence of tibiotalar arthritic changes (stage IV osteonecrosis).[10]

RELEVANT ANATOMY

Several branches of the dorsalis pedis artery may act as pedicles for vascularized bone grafts. Potential harvest sites include the cuboid, the medial cuneiform, or the lateral cuneiform. Harvesting from the cuboid allows for the largest grafts, measuring about 2 × 1 cm on average, and the longest pedicle, averaging 4 cm in length (**Fig. 1**).[11] For this reason, we prefer use of cuboid grafts for the treatment of talar osteonecrosis, which often requires a larger graft.

The primary blood supply to the cuboid is from the proximal lateral tarsal artery, which originates from the dorsalis pedis artery at the level of the talar head or neck. From its origin, it travels distally and laterally toward the cuboid. It gives off a variable number of branches before reaching the cuboid, where it provides 8 to 20 nutrient vessels to the dorsum of the cuboid.[11]

SURGICAL TECHNIQUE

This procedure is performed supine with a bump under the ipsilateral hip such that the foot points to the ceiling. Regional anesthesia is advised, because it aides in preventing vasospasm of the delicate arteries supplying the tarsal bones. A thigh tourniquet is used.

Approach

A standard anterior approach to the ankle is used proximally, and extended distally by curving laterally over the cuboid.

- Care is taken to protect the superficial peroneal nerve distally.
- The extensor retinaculum is opened over the extensor hallucis longus (EHL) tendon.
- The dorsalis pedis artery is identified between the EHL tendon and the extensor digitorum longus tendon.

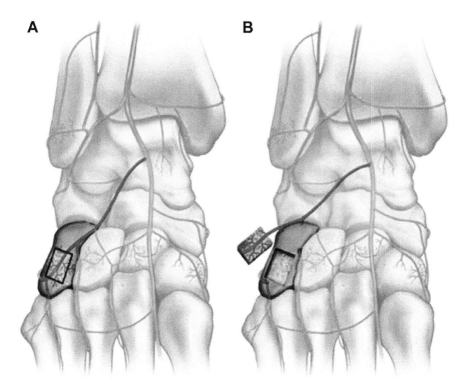

Fig. 1. The primary blood supply to the cuboid, from the proximal lateral tarsal artery, is illustrated (*A*). The resulting pedicle graft (*B*) has sufficient excursion to reach any site along the neck of the talus. (*From* Nunley JA, Hamid KS. Vascularized pedicle bone-grafting from the cuboid for talar osteonecrosis. J Bone Joint Surg Am 2017;99(10):848–54; with permission.)

- The proximal lateral tarsal artery is identified at the level of the talar head or neck, where it branches off laterally from the dorsalis pedis artery.
- The artery is dissected from proximal to distal, as it travels laterally under the muscle bellies of the extensor hallucis brevis and extensor digitorum brevis (EDB). Care should be taken to preserve the lateral branch of the deep peroneal nerve, which lies alongside the artery.
- Attention is then turned to the distal aspect of the incision, where the EDB muscle belly is elevated off the cuboid, starting at its lateral edge and progressing medially. While elevating the muscle, the pedicle artery comes into view (**Fig. 2**).

Harvesting the Vascularized Graft

- With the pedicle artery now fully exposed, small (0.2 mm) Kirschner wires are placed at the corners of the planned graft harvest and then checked under fluoroscopy to ensure that the harvest does not violate any articular surfaces.
- Hemoclips are used to ligate the various branches of the artery to enable graft excursion.
- Straight followed by curved osteotomes are used to harvest the bone underlying the nutrient vessels supplied by the pedicle artery. The graft is mobilized and passed under the EDB into the anterior aspect of the incision (**Fig. 3**).
- Papaverine may be used to prevent vasospasm when manipulating the pedicle.

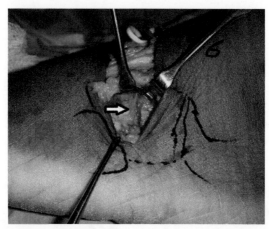

Fig. 2. In the lateral aspect of the incision, the EDB muscle belly is retracted dorsally to expose the pedicle artery (*arrow*) overlying the cuboid.

Preparation of the Talus

Before insertion of the graft, the area of talar osteonecrosis is drilled and debrided to remove all necrotic bone.

- At the level of the ankle joint, the neurovascular bundle is retracted laterally with the EHL tendon and a longitudinal capsulotomy is made to expose the tibiotalar joint.
- A guide pin is inserted into the area of osteonecrosis from anterior to posterior, starting at the talar neck-dome junction to avoid damage to the articular surface. Fluoroscopy is used to confirm an appropriate trajectory (**Fig. 4**).
- Using cannulated drills, the guide pin is sequentially overdrilled to open the area of necrotic bone (**Fig. 5**).

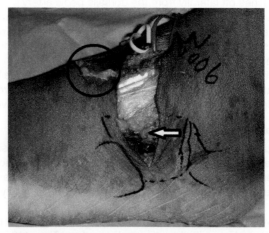

Fig. 3. The pedicle graft (*circled*) is shown, after it has been passed under the EDB, extensor digitorum longus, and EHL tendons to reach the talus. The EDB muscle belly, uninjured, now overlies the harvest site (*arrow*).

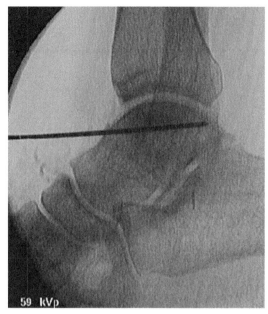

Fig. 4. A guide pin is placed into the center of the area of talar osteonecrosis, starting at the talar head-neck junction.

- Curettes and/or a burr set at low torque may be used to remove any remaining necrotic bone, taking care to avoid any damage to the joint.
- The resulting cavity may be filled with contrast medium and examined under multiple fluoroscopic views to ensure adequate removal of necrotic bone and debris (**Fig. 6**).

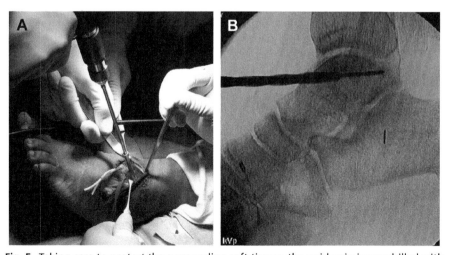

Fig. 5. Taking care to protect the surrounding soft tissues, the guide pin is overdrilled with sequential cannulated drills (*A*). Fluoroscopy is used to ensure adequate penetration of the area of osteonecrosis (*B*).

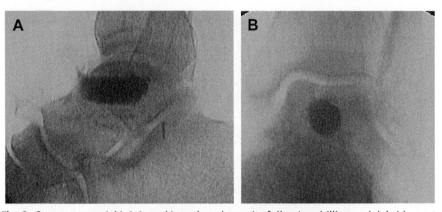

Fig. 6. Contrast material is injected into the talar cavity following drilling and debridement. Lateral (*A*) and anteroposterior (*B*) fluoroscopic views are used to ensure adequate resection of necrotic bone.

Insertion of the Vascularized Graft

- The vascularized bone graft and the talar cavity are contoured to allow for a close interference fit.
- The graft is carefully inserted into the talar cavity. No fixation is used to avoid damage to the blood supply.
- The tourniquet is released to ensure that there is blood flow to the graft. The ankle is ranged to ensure that there is no tension on the pedicle.

Postoperative Protocol

- A short leg splint is applied and patients are instructed to maintain nonweightbearing status.
- At 2 weeks, sutures are removed and a short leg cast is applied.
- At 4 weeks, the cast is removed and range of motion and strengthening exercises for the ankle are initiated. Patients remain nonweightbearing in a removable boot.
- At 3 months, radiographs are taken and patients are allowed to start gradually advancing weightbearing while using a patellar tendon-bearing brace. Patients are instructed to wear the brace until 1 year postoperatively to offload the ankle.
- At 1 year, an MRI scan may be performed to assess for any changes in articular congruity and/or bone marrow signal compared with preoperative MRI.

OUTCOMES

The only outcomes reported in the literature are from small case series, all with differing methodologies. We reported on a series of 13 patients treated with vascularized bone grafting from the cuboid for talar osteonecrosis, using the technique described previously. Over a mean 6 years follow-up, 11 patients (85%) required no additional surgery for talar osteonecrosis. These patients had significant improvement in patient-reported outcome scores. Two patients who failed treatment underwent total ankle replacement.[10] Improvement on MRI in patients treated with this technique is impressive, as illustrated in **Fig. 7**.

Other authors have described using a vascularized cuneiform bone flap, reporting good or excellent results in more than 80% of patients.[8,9] In a series of 24 patients

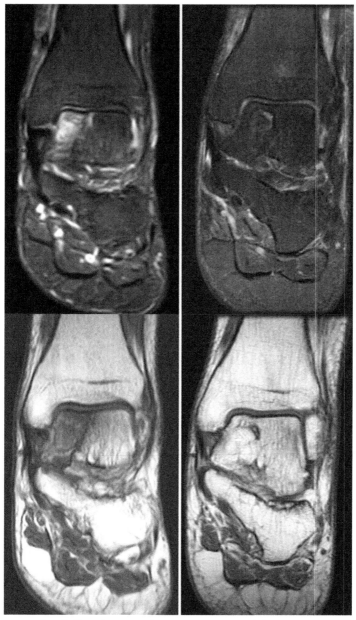

Fig. 7. Preoperative (*left*) and 15 months postoperative (*right*) coronal MRI images for a 42-year-old patient with osteonecrosis of the talus treated with a vascularized pedicle graft from the cuboid. Fat-suppressed T2-weighted images (*top*) and T1-weighted images (*bottom*) are shown.

who received either a cuneiform or cuboid vascularized graft, 83% of patients had a good or excellent result.[9] Yu and colleagues[8] augmented the cuneiform bone flap with cancellous iliac crest autograft in 20 patients, with 90% good or excellent results.

COMPARISON WITH OTHER JOINT-SPARING SURGICAL TECHNIQUES

Joint-sparing treatment options include core decompression and either vascularized or nonvascularized bone grafting.[2] Delanois and colleagues[6] and Marulanda and colleagues[5] reported successful outcomes in 91% of patients treated with core decompression. Mont and colleagues[7] reported good or excellent outcomes in 82% of patients treated with core decompression. A case report noted good outcomes in a patient with stage II disease treated with both core decompression and an internal bone stimulator.[12] We have also had success using core decompression when the entire talar body is involved.

Few studies have compared joint-sparing treatment methods. Hernigou and colleagues[4] compared patients who underwent core decompression alone with those who underwent core decompression with iliac crest bone marrow aspirate concentrate (BMAC) injection. Over a mean 17 years follow-up, 80% of patients who received BMAC had successful treatment, compared with 29% who underwent core decompression alone, with failure defined as need for arthrodesis. Moreover, when arthrodesis was required, the patients who received BMAC had a higher fusion rate (100% vs 73%).[4]

Of note, all patients in the previously mentioned studies had stage I or II disease, unlike the vascularized graft studies, which also included patients with stage III disease. Therefore, direct comparisons between treatment methods are difficult to make.

SUMMARY

Vascularized bone grafting for talar osteonecrosis has had encouraging outcomes in small case series. Microvascular expertise is not required to perform this procedure. It represents a good treatment option for patients with stage II and III changes and minimal subchondral collapse. Combining use of a vascularized pedicle graft with additional augments, including cancellous iliac crest bone graft or BMAC, may confer additional success. However, data remain limited, with few comparative studies to guide treatment.

REFERENCES

1. Arlet J, Ficat R. [Forage-biopsie de la tête fémorale dans l'ostéonécrose primitive. Observations histo-pathologiques portent sur nuit forages]. Rev Rhum 1964;31: 257–64.
2. Gross CE, Sershon RA, Frank JM, et al. Treatment of osteonecrosis of the talus. JBJS Rev 2016;4(7). https://doi.org/10.2106/JBJS.RVW.15.00087.
3. Gross CE, Haughom B, Chahal J, et al. Treatments for osteonecrosis of the talus: a systematic review. Foot Ankle Spec 2014;7(5):387–97.
4. Hernigou P, Dubory A, Flouzat Lachaniette CH, et al. Stem cell therapy in early post-traumatic talus osteonecrosis. Int Orthop 2018. [Epub ahead of print].
5. Marulanda GA, McGrath MS, Ulrich SD, et al. Percutaneous drilling for the treatment of atraumatic osteonecrosis of the ankle. J Foot Ankle Surg 2010;49(1):20–4.
6. Delanois RE, Mont MA, Yoon TR, et al. Atraumatic osteonecrosis of the talus. J Bone Joint Surg Am 1998;80(4):529–36.
7. Mont MA, Schon LC, Hungerford MW, et al. Osteonecrosis of the talus treated by core decompression. J Bone Joint Surg Br 1996;78(5):827–30.
8. Yu XG, Zhao DW, Sun Q, et al. Treatment of non-traumatic avascular talar necrosis by transposition of vascularized cuneiform bone flap plus iliac cancellous bone grafting. Zhonghua Yi Xue Za Zhi 2010;90(15):1035–8.

9. Zhang Y, Liu Y, Jiang Y. Treatment of osteonecrosis of talus with vascularized bone graft. Zhongguo Xiu Fu Chong Jian Wai Ke Za Zhi 1998;12(5):285–7.
10. Nunley JA, Hamid KS. Vascularized pedicle bone-grafting from the cuboid for talar osteonecrosis: results of a novel salvage procedure. J Bone Joint Surg Am 2017;99(10):848–54.
11. Gilbert BJ, Horst F, Nunley JA. Potential donor rotational bone grafts using vascular territories in the foot and ankle. J Bone Joint Surg Am 2004;86-A(9): 1857–73.
12. Holmes GB Jr, Wydra F, Hellman M, et al. A unique treatment for talar osteonecrosis: placement of an internal bone stimulator: a case report. JBJS Case Connect 2015;5(1):e4–5.

Ankle Arthrodesis for Talar Avascular Necrosis and Arthrodesis Nonunion

Jonathon D. Backus, MD*, Daniel L. Ocel, MD

KEYWORDS

- Avascular necrosis • Osteonecrosis • Talar collapse • Arthrodesis • Nonunion

KEY POINTS

- 75% of Talar avascular necrosis (AVN) is associated with trauma, and in particular, talar neck fractures.
- Revascularization of the talus can take up to 36 months by creeping substitution.
- Prolonged non–weight bearing, partial weight bearing, and bracing have been used for conservative treatment but have not been shown to prevent collapse or improve outcomes.
- Tibiotalar arthrodesis, subtalar arthrodesis, and tibiotalocalcaneal arthrodesis are all potential options for treating late-stage talar AVN based on patient examination, imaging, and selective joint injections.
- Principles of arthrodesis include the removal of any necrotic bone; the addition of autograft, allograft, and various biologic augments for incorporation; and instrumentation that maintains appropriate rigidity, compression, and alignment.

INTRODUCTION

Avascular necrosis (AVN) of the talus is a complex and challenging condition for clinicians and patients. Symptoms include pain, deformity, and at times complete loss of the ankle joint or significant arthritic changes that result in impaired ambulation. AVN of the talus is believed associated with ankle trauma in 75% of cases.[1] Talar neck fractures are the most common cause of talar AVN, and its incidence increases with severity of the original injury. Modern talar AVN rates are 9.8%, 27.4%, 53.4%, and 48.0% for Hawkins types I to IV fractures, respectively.[2] Other causes of talar AVN include corticosteroid use, Addison disease, Cushing disease, alcoholism, chronic

Dr D.L. Ocel is a paid Consultant for Articulus Bio and Ossur. Dr J.D. Backus has nothing to disclose.
Cornerstone Orthopaedics and Sports Medicine, 3 Superior Drive, Suite 225, Superior, CO 80027, USA
* Corresponding author.
E-mail address: jon.backus@gmail.com

pancreatitis, sickle cell disease, peripheral vascular disease, chronic renal failure, lupus, and iatrogenic surgical complications.[3]

As Horst and colleagues[4] suggested, it is important to differentiate AVN into early and late stages for the basis of treatment. In the early stages of AVN, conservative treatment and joint sparing procedures, such as bone grafting and decompression, are possible to decrease symptoms and stop the natural history of the condition. Treatment of late stages of AVN (greater than 12 months) of the talus is limited and often requires arthrodesis, arthroplasty, or, in extreme cases, talectomy. The purpose of this article is to review the arthrodesis options for the later stages of talar AVN.

CONSERVATIVE TREATMENT

Revascularization of the talus occurs via creeping substitution and can take up to 36 months.[5] During this period of revascularization, the main concern of clinicians is to prevent talar collapse. Traditionally, patients were instructed to remain non–weight bearing until both fracture healing and revascularization occurred.[6,7] As can be imagined, tolerance of and compliance with non–weight bearing or limited weight bearing for 3 years is low and this treatment has not been demonstrated to prevent talar collapse (**Fig. 1**). Even the investigators of the study that defined the period of creeping substitution concluded that there was no increased risk of collapse with weight bearing on an avascular talus.[5] Nevertheless, there is another group of clinicians who have advocated for partial weight bearing and protective bracing.[8–10] Unfortunately, none of these conservative treatment modalities has been proved to decrease the risk of poor outcomes.[11] In a recent systematic review, 33% of patients treated conservatively ultimately needed a surgical procedure, with an average of 95 months' follow-up.[12]

Another conservative modality includes the use of extracorporeal shock wave therapy (ECSWT) to stimulate revascularization of the talus. In a level I study, Zhai and colleagues[13] compared ECSWT with physical therapy alone in 34 patients. They found

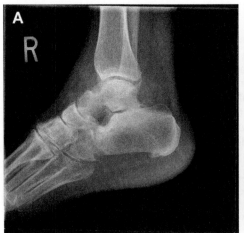
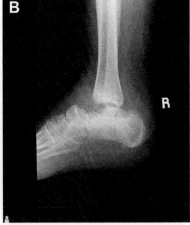

Fig. 1. (A) Avascular talus before collapse in a 46-year-old man status-post talonavicular and subtalar dislocation that was initially treated conservatively. He developed subtalar arthritis and was scheduled for a subtalar arthrodesis. (B) Talus collapsed 28 months from the initial injury and was identified at a preoperative appointment. Subsequent work-up was negative for infection, diabetes, peripheral neuropathy, and syringomyelia.

significant improvement in American Orthopaedic Foot & Ankle Society (AOFAS) hind-foot scores and visual analog scale (VAS) scores for pain compared with physical therapy alone at 18 months. Furthermore, only 1 patient required arthrodesis in this study. Although these results are promising, to the authors' knowledge no other confirmatory reports of this modality for AVN exist in the literature.

The unpredictable pain response to an avascular talus is the primary source of confusion related to the issue of conservative treatment. It has often been observed that radiographic findings and pain do not necessarily correlate. Therefore, some investigators advocate for using pain as a guideline for treatment.[4] Painless AVN can be treated with non–weight bearing, bracing, or observation, as discussed previously. Painful, early AVN can be treated with bone grafting[4,14–16] and/or core decompression.[17–19] Because of the partially subjective nature of this treatment algorithm, many patients progress to the later stages of AVN, where salvage operations are necessary.

SURGICAL TREATMENT OF LATE AVASCULAR NECROSIS

In cases of late AVN, patient and clinician are often left with few treatment options. Because talectomy is rarely performed and is noted to have poor results,[20,21] this article focuses on the array of arthrodesis options to treat this condition. Unfortunately, for patients, tibiotalar (TT) arthrodesis, subtalar arthrodesis, talonavicular arthrodesis, triple arthrodesis, and tibiotalocalcaneal (TTC) arthrodesis all result in some form of gait abnormality. It is also widely believed that fusion will lead to adjacent joints to become arthritic overtime,[22,23] potentially increasing the likelihood of needing further operations. Given that most cases of AVN are the result of talar neck fractures, there is an additional element of posttraumatic arthritis. It is believed that TT and subtalar posttraumatic arthritis occurs in 30% and 81% of talar neck fractures, respectively.[2] This, in conjunction with younger patient age, makes arthrodesis an undesirable but necessary operation to treat pain and potentially talar collapse.

TIBIOTALAR ARTHRODESIS

TT arthrodesis is a good option for pain control in the setting of isolated ankle symptoms and minimal talar collapse. There are various techniques available to achieve a TT fusion but all require sufficient bone stock to hold adequate fixation after débridement of the avascular bone. The ankle should be fused in neutral dorsiflexion, 0° to 5° of hindfoot valgus and 5° to 10° of external rotation, for optimal functional results.[24] Traditional open TT arthrodesis can occur through an anterior, transfibular, or posterior approach as long as congruent opposing cancellous bone is rigidly compressed and fixed. The decision of which approach to take depends on surgeon comfort, status of the soft tissue envelope, and location of prior incisions. Both cancellous and structural autograft or allograft bone grafting should be used as needed to fill in any voids from avascular bone or subchondral cysts. The outcomes of open isolated ankle arthrodesis for talar AVN are not well reported. This is likely because many cases of late-stage talar AVN require fusion of the subtalar joint as well. Kitaoka and Patzer[25] reported favorable results for arthrodesis union, but only 3 of these patients had an isolated TT arthrodesis.

In cases of no talar collapse and minimal deformity, arthroscopic ankle arthrodesis is a viable alternative. This can be achieved through the anteromedial and anterolateral portals with a combination of arthroscopic shavers, burs, rasps, and curettes. Some investigators add a posterolateral portal to help further prepare the joint and remove cartilage or extend the portal incisions for a miniopen approach. Fixation is achieved through percutaneous screw fixation, and screw orientation and number varies per surgeon preference. Arthroscopic ankle fusion offers the benefit of decreased blood loss, preservation of the soft tissue envelope and vasculature, quicker union time, and increased union rate.[26] Kendal and colleagues[27] reported good results and fusion in all 15 patients of their series with arthroscopic ankle arthrodesis for talar AVN. Only 3 patients had continued pain, and symptoms resolved with a subsequent subtalar arthrodesis.

Another form of TT arthrodesis includes the Blair arthrodesis where the talar body is removed and a distal tibial inlay bone graft is inserted to restore height (**Fig. 2**).[28] The original procedure had a high nonunion rate at 28% and has been modified extensively with the addition of various internal fixation devices.[28–30] Van Bergeyk and colleagues[29] and Lionberger and colleagues[28] reported 71% and 80% union rates, respectively, with their versions of the modified Blair arthrodesis, making union rates nearly comparable to fusion in non-AVN cases.

SUBTALAR ARTHRODESIS

Subtalar arthrodesis for talar AVN with isolated subtalar symptoms and no talar collapse is a viable treatment modality. Unfortunately, this situation is rare because the TT joint is usually symptomatic. Much like the TT joint, this procedure can be performed both open or arthroscopically. It is important to débride osteonecrotic bone

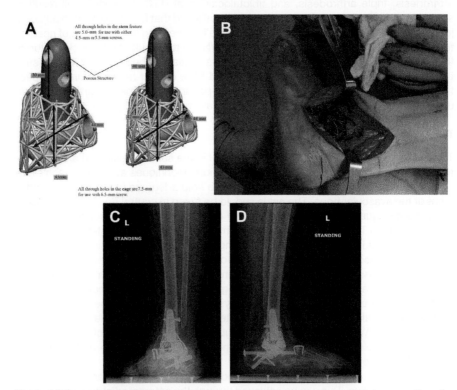

Fig. 2. (*A*) Preoperative planned model for custom 3-D cage implant. (*B*) Intraoperative picture of a custom 3-D cage implant being inserted through a lateral transfibular approach. Intraoperative (*C*) anteroposterior and (*D*) lateral fluoroscopic images of implanted 3-D cage in the same patient. (*Courtesy of* David B. Hahn, MD, Denver, CO.)

and restore alignment to 5° to 10° of hindfoot valgus[31] during this procedure. Fixation is usually achieved with various numbers and types of cannulated or solid screws. In a large series of subtalar arthrodeses with an average of over 4 years' follow-up, AOFAS hindfoot scores increased from 24 to 70 and union was achieved in 84% of the 184 patients[32]; 42% had evidence of 2 mm or greater of avascular bone and all 30 non-unions occurred in this group. The investigators also identified smoking and prior non-unions as risk factors for nonunion.

With minimal talar collapse, subtalar arthrodesis may aid in revascularization of the talus through creeping substitution. This could allow for a total ankle arthroplasty to be used to treat TT symptoms. Although AVN of the talus is usually a relative contraindication for a total ankle, Lee and colleagues[33] have published 2 successful cases in patients where revascularization was proved through radionuclide bone scanning. Furthermore, Devalia and colleagues[34] describe a novel technique where ankle replacement was staged for talar AVN an average of 9.5 months after a subtalar arthrodesis in 7 patients. They had good results with increased AOFAS, Western Ontario and McMaster Universities Osteoarthritis Index, and 36-Item Short Form Health Survey (SF-36) scores after surgery, and 5 patients were satisfied at 3 years' follow-up. Two patients had asymptomatic radiographic evidence of talar component subsidence.

TIBIOTALOCALCANEAL FUSION WITH 3-D IMPLANTS

TTC arthrodesis is often necessary for late-stage AVN and is discussed in detail in James R. Lachman and Samuel B. Adams' article, "Tibiotalar-Calcaneal Arthrodesis for Severe Talar Avascular Necrosis," in this issue. Nevertheless, some emerging technologies designed to treat this challenging condition are discussed briefly. New to the treatment arsenal for hindfoot fusion for AVN of the talus, in both primary and revision cases, is the utilization of 3-D titanium cage truss systems in addition to talar replacements (see **Fig. 2**). These new systems use CT modeling and 3-D printing to create strong porous structures that can be packed with bone graft or biologic adjuvants (4WEB Medical, Frisco, Texas, and Additive Orthopaedics, Little Silver, New Jersey). Unlike allograft inlays, these greatly decrease the chances of reabsorption and subsequent collapse of the graft tissue during bone incorporation. Case reports of patient-specific 3-D printed cages have been shown to have early success.[35–37] In discussions with the few surgeons currently incorporating this technology into their practice, the prevailing belief is that these implants potentially may aid the foot and ankle surgeon in dealing with the severe altered anatomy of the hindfoot, bone loss, and other confounding factors complicating AVN treatment. In doing so, this may bolster the armamentarium in the realm of preservation of the lower extremity in cases that otherwise would progress to amputation. Unfortunately, because these implants are new to the market, no substantial research is available to date. Further studies are needed in this regard to prove their viability.

OTHER HINDFOOT ARTHRODESIS

Talonavicular arthrodesis, triple arthodesis, and pantalar arthrodesis have been proposed by others for the treatment of avsacular necrosis.[38] In the authors' experience, indications for these procedures are rare and no case series discussing them have been published for talar AVN. Nevertheless, in situations with isolated talonavicular pain, calcaneocuboid pain, or significant hindfoot deformity, these options can be considered.

OUTCOMES

Outcomes of hindfoot arthrodesis with talar AVN for each isolated arthrodesis are limited and many investigators have combined them with TTC fusion procedures. A recent systematic review of 19 studies found that the overall evidence regarding treatment of AVN is lacking and nearly impossible to pool.[12] In the 6 articles on arthrodesis, there was limited consensus on outcomes measures and modalities used to determine union. Furthermore, all studies were retrospective case series. Dennison and colleagues,[30] Devries and colleagues,[39] and Urquhart and colleagues[40] reported union at an average of 8 months. Lionberger and colleagues[28] reported 80% union at 3 months. Van Bergeyk and colleagues[29] reported union in 71% of patients at 4 months. Furthermore, in the Van Bergeyk and colleagues study, postoperative AOFAS hindfoot scores were an average of 67; SF-36 physical score was an average of 46 for the physical component and 61 for the mental component; and postoperative VAS score was an average of 7.1 for pain.[29] Kitaoka and Patzer[25] found that 36.8% of patients had excellent results, 31.6% had good results, 15.8% had fair results, and 15.8% had poor results using their own criteria. They also concluded that those patients who were younger than 30 years old, weighed less than 76.5 kg, and did not have previous operations had better outcomes. Urquhart reported that Mazur scores improved from 27.5 to 86 in patients who fused.[40]

In the same systematic review, the pooled delayed union rate was 32% and infection rate was 16%.[12] Kitaoka and Patzer[25] reported a nonunion rate of 18%. They also had reoperations in 15% of their series, 7% had repeat arthrodesis attempts, and 1 (2%) patient required a below-knee amputation.

In Devries and colleagues'[39] study of TTC arthrodesis with a hindfoot nail, the complication rate was 14% for hardware complications, 14% for necessary irrigation and débridement, and 14% for stress fractures.

INTREPID DYNAMIC EXOSKELETAL ORTHOSIS BRACING

Another preoperative and postoperative option for treatment of AVN of the talus is the use of newer dynamic ankle-foot orthoses. Previously, individuals with either salvaged lower extremities from high-energy trauma or posttraumatic arthritis had limited bracing options. Classic braces, such as rigid and articulated ankle-foot orthoses, significantly reduced triplane hindfoot motion and many patients who used these devices were unable to return to any significant activity level.[41] With the advent of dynamic response system orthoses (ie, Intrepid Dynamic Exoskeletal Orthosis [IDEO]/ ExoSym, Hanger Clinic, Gig Harbor, Washington, and PHAT, Phat Brace, Des Moines, Iowa), clinicians have been able to delay further surgical interventions and improve performance capabilities in younger patients with significant deformity or posttraumatic arthritis (**Fig. 3**). In a comparison of the effects of orthosis design on functional performance, the IDEO brace significantly improved performance on selective measures in individuals considering amputation.[42] In the authors' experience, many of the individuals with this condition would like to return to more substantive activities, such as running. The use of IDEO bracing has been shown beneficial in the acquisition of this capability in the high-functioning individual.[43]

NONUNIONS

The true incidence of hindfoot fusion nonunion is unknown, because many studies have not included advanced imaging to confirm bridging bone. As discussed previously, the delayed union rate in a systematic review for all hindfoot fusions in AVN

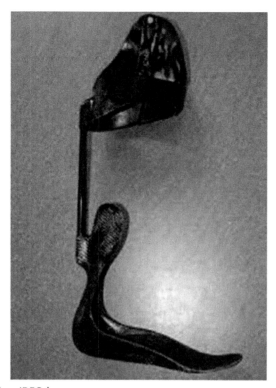

Fig. 3. Picture of an IDEO brace.

cases was 32%,[12] but 1 study reported a nonunion rate as high as 29%.[29] Even in cases without talar AVN, hindfoot arthrodesis nonunion but can be upward of 28% in ankle fusions[44] and 48% in TTC arthrodesis.[45] Nonunion is more common in patients that are compromised by tobacco use, peripheral neuropathy, nutritionally deficiency, diabetes, and peripheral vascular disease. (**Fig. 4**).[32,45] During preoperative counseling with patients, discussion regarding expectations, compliance, and modulation of other variables is imperative.

It is also important to ensure that the proper technical aspects of surgery are thoroughly followed: removal of all nonviable bone, cartilage, and fibrous tissue; minimal soft tissue dissection; and identification and eradication of infection and appropriate fixation. Rigid fixation is of utmost importance regardless of type of fixation chosen (cannulated screws, locking plates, blade plates, intramedullary devices, and external fixation).

Biological augmentation of healing is an essential adjunct to the surgical aspects of nonunion treatment. Clinicians are able to manipulate bone biology to promote healing with 3 types of bioactive agents: osteoconductive (allografts), osteoinductive (autografts, bone morphogenic proteins, and platelet-derived growth factor), and osteogenic (autografts, bone marrow aspirate concentrate, and platelet-rich plasma) materials.[46] Osteoconductive agents function to provide a scaffold matrix for cells to infiltrate prompting bone growth across this scaffold. Osteoinductive agents stimulate nondifferentiated cells to convert to osteoblasts and other bone-forming cells whereas osteogenic materials provide cells that can actually produce bone. Although specific product use is outside the scope of this review, the authors often consider the

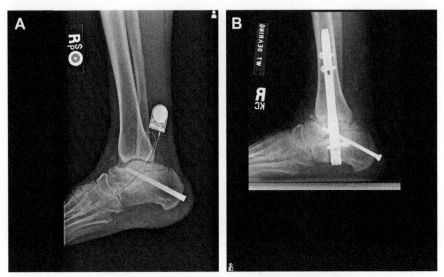

Fig. 4. (*A*) Lateral radiograph of a 48-year-old woman with diabetes and peripheral neuropathy who is status post–talar neck fracture and partial talar collapse who underwent subtalar arthrodesis and bone stimulator implantation by another surgeon. Unfortunately, she went on to a painful arthrodesis nonunion. (*B*) Lateral radiograph of the same patient 4 months post-TTC arthrodesis with recombinant human platelet-derived growth factor bone graft and bone autograft who developed another nonunion despite cast immobilization and 3 months of non–weight bearing. Subsequent endocrine work-up was negative for nutritional deficiency or hormonal imbalance. This illustrates how challenging fusions can be in patients with an avascular talus.

addition of an osteogenic and/or osteoinductive product or bone graft to aid in the treatment of nonunion cases.

Both internal and external device bone stimulation can also be considered in the treatment of nonunion. These include pulsed electromagnetic field (PEMF), low-intensity pulsed ultrasound (LIPUS), and implantable direct current (DC) devices. The exact mechanism of PEMF and LIPUS is not completely understood; however, both seem to stimulate healing through transformation growth factor β (TGF-β)–mediated differentiation of fibrocartilage cells as well as a stimulatory effect directly on the osteoblast.[47] In a study by Saltzman and colleagues,[48] however, the investigators used PEMF in the treatment of 19 cases of delayed union after hindfoot arthrodesis and found success in only 5 of 19 patients. LIPUS has seen increased attention with regard to the treatment of at-risk delayed unions and nonunions.[49] The high cost of utilization of these units presents a barrier to usage; however, Jones and colleagues[50] in a prospective comparative study that evaluated both clinical and radiographic healing in the primary subtalar arthrodesis demonstrated 100% healing rate, decreased union time, and improved clinical function compared with the control group. Implantable DC (I-DC) bone stimulation has shown positive outcomes with regard to the treatment of hindfoot fusion in several studies (see **Fig. 4**).[51,52] Complications did arise with regard to cable breakage, superficial breakdown of wound, and revision surgery to remove batteries. Midis and Conti[53] did demonstrate successful fusion in 10 of 10 patients treated for aseptic nonunion of ankle fusion with revision arthrodesis and placement of an I-DC unit.

DISCUSSION

The evidence for treatment of AVN of the talus is lacking. To the authors' knowledge, only 1 level I study has been performed, and this focuses on ECSWT for nonoperative treatment.[13] A majority of reports are level IV studies, where a substantial amount of reporting bias can be assumed. Simply put, even the most honest of surgeons are not likely to publish negative results critical of their practice. But in fairness to the profession, it is extraordinarily time-consuming, expensive, and difficult to obtain Institutional Review Board approval, ensure contributing surgeons maintain clinical equipoise, and execute level I studies on surgical outcomes. Furthermore, in the current social climate, many patients are not keen to participate in random assignment treatment. Nevertheless, more high-level studies are needed to help aid the community in advancing treatment of this challenging and often frustrating condition.

In the authors' experience of treating late-stage symptomatic talar AVN, focusing on the joints that are involved with the process is needed, that is, talonavicular, subtalar, TT, or both. This can be determined at least in part by focal diagnostic injections in the involved joints[54] and a thorough history and physical examination. In addition, the provider needs to be keenly aware of whether or not a patient suffers from focally isolated involvement of the talus or diffuse AVN throughout the body itself. Focally involved AVN that is symptomatic may be treated with joint-preserving procedures, which are not the focus of this review. Diffuse symptomatic AVN usually results in joint-sacrificing arthrodesis procedures that treat pain but ultimately limit function. This highlights the importance of advanced imaging that is routinely obtained in the treatment of AVN. TT, subtalar, and TTC arthrodesis all should be considered in the salvage treatment of Talar AVN. The keys to successful fusion, as in any arthrodesis procedure, include the removal of any necrotic bone; the addition of autograft, allograft, and various biologic augments for incorporation; and instrumentation that maintains appropriate compression and alignment. The newer 3-D printed implants and arthroplasty components may provide improved treatment results in the future. Furthermore, the newer dynamic braces also can be used before or after an arthrodesis operation to help high-functioning patients try to resume some of their activities. More investigation is necessary in determining the viability of these new implants and orthoses for talar AVN.

Many investigators consider arthrodesis a salvage operation and last resort for talar AVN. This is amplified by the fact that this condition is posttraumatic and often effects younger patients. Yet, as Kitaoka and Patzer[25] concluded, 60% of patients without previous operations go on to have improved fusion outcomes compared with patients with previous surgeries. It is, therefore, important to remember that pain control is balanced with function and often both cannot be achieved simultaneously. Perhaps clinicians should shift their focus and counseling to explain these procedures as reconstructive options rather than salvage procedures. As with all medicine, it is important to tailor treatment plans to the individual and set appropriate expectations.

REFERENCES

1. Metzger MJ, Levin JS, Clancy JT. Talar neck fractures and rates of avascular necrosis. J Foot Ankle Surg 1999;38(2):154–62.
2. Dodd A, Lefaivre KA. Outcomes of talar neck fractures: a systematic review and meta-analysis. J Orthop Trauma 2015;29(5):210–5.
3. Hermus JP. Osteonecrosis of the talus after talonavicular arthrodesis: a case report and review of the literature. J Foot Ankle Surg 2011;50(3):343–6.

4. Horst F, Gilbert BJ, Nunley JA. Avascular necrosis of the talus: current treatment options. Foot Ankle Clin 2004;9(4):757–73.
5. Penny JN, Davis LA. Fractures and fracture-dislocations of the neck of the talus. J Trauma 1980;20(12):1029–37.
6. Adelaar RS. The treatment of complex fractures of the talus. Orthop Clin North Am 1989;20(4):691–707.
7. Canale ST. Fractures of the neck of the talus. Orthopedics 1990;13(10):1105–15.
8. Comfort TH, Behrens F, Gaither DW, et al. Long-term results of displaced talar neck fractures. Clin Orthop Relat Res 1985;(199):81–7.
9. Grob D, Simpson LA, Weber BG, et al. Operative treatment of displaced talus fractures. Clin Orthop Relat Res 1985;(199):88–96.
10. Szyszkowitz R, Reschauer R, Seggl W. Eighty-five talus fractures treated by ORIF with five to eight years of follow-up study of 69 patients. Clin Orthop Relat Res 1985;(199):97–107.
11. Henderson RC. Posttraumatic necrosis of the talus: the Hawkins sign versus magnetic resonance imaging. J Orthop Trauma 1991;5(1):96–9.
12. Gross CE, Haughom B, Chahal J, et al. Treatments for avascular necrosis of the talus: a systematic review. Foot Ankle Spec 2014;7(5):387–97.
13. Zhai L, Sun N, Zhang BQ, et al. Effect of liquid-electric extracorporeal shock wave on treating traumatic avascular necrosis of talus. Journal of Clinical Rehabilitative Tissue Engineering Research 2010;14(17):3135–8.
14. Doi K, Hattori Y. Vascularized bone graft from the supracondylar region of the femur. Microsurgery 2009;29(5):379–84.
15. Hussl H, Sailer R, Daniaux H, et al. Revascularization of a partially necrotic talus with a vascularized bone graft from the iliac crest. Arch Orthop Trauma Surg 1989;108(1):27–9.
16. Kenwright J, Taylor RG. Major injuries of the talus. J Bone Joint Surg Br 1970; 52(1):36–48.
17. Marulanda GA, McGrath MS, Ulrich SD, et al. Percutaneous drilling for the treatment of atraumatic osteonecrosis of the ankle. J Foot Ankle Surg 2010;49(1): 20–4.
18. Delanois RE, Mont MA, Yoon TR, et al. Atraumatic osteonecrosis of the talus. J Bone Joint Surg Am 1998;80(4):529–36.
19. Mont MA, Schon LC, Hungerford MW, et al. Avascular necrosis of the talus treated by core decompression. J Bone Joint Surg Br 1996;78(5):827–30.
20. Coltart WD. Aviator's astragalus. J Bone Joint Surg Br 1952;34-B(4):545–66.
21. Hawkins LG. Fractures of the neck of the talus. J Bone Joint Surg Am 1970;52(5): 991–1002.
22. Ebalard M, Le Henaff G, Sigonney G, et al. Risk of osteoarthritis secondary to partial or total arthrodesis of the subtalar and midtarsal joints after a minimum follow-up of 10 years. Orthop Traumatol Surg Res 2014;100(4 Suppl):S231–7.
23. Coester LM, Saltzman CL, Leupold J, et al. Long-term results following ankle arthrodesis for post-traumatic arthritis. J Bone Joint Surg Am 2001;83-A(2): 219–28.
24. Buck P, Morrey BF, Chao EY. The optimum position of arthrodesis of the ankle. A gait study of the knee and ankle. J Bone Joint Surg Am 1987;69(7):1052–62.
25. Kitaoka HB, Patzer GL. Arthrodesis for the treatment of arthrosis of the ankle and osteonecrosis of the talus. J Bone Joint Surg Am 1998;80(3):370–9.
26. Horst F, Nunley JA 2nd. Ankle arthrodesis. J Surg Orthop Adv 2004;13(2):81–90.
27. Kendal AR, Cooke P, Sharp R. Arthroscopic ankle fusion for avascular necrosis of the talus. Foot Ankle Int 2015;36(5):591–7.

28. Lionberger DR, Bishop JO, Tullos HS. The modified Blair fusion. Foot Ankle 1982; 3(1):60–2.
29. Van Bergeyk A, Stotler W, Beals T, et al. Functional outcome after modified Blair tibiotalar arthrodesis for talar osteonecrosis. Foot Ankle Int 2003;24(10):765–70.
30. Dennison MG, Pool RD, Simonis RB, et al. Tibiocalcaneal fusion for avascular necrosis of the talus. J Bone Joint Surg Br 2001;83(2):199–203.
31. Jastifer JR, Gustafson PA, Gorman RR. Subtalar arthrodesis alignment: the effect on ankle biomechanics. Foot Ankle Int 2013;34(2):244–50.
32. Easley ME, Trnka HJ, Schon LC, et al. Isolated subtalar arthrodesis. J Bone Joint Surg Am 2000;82(5):613–24.
33. Lee KB, Cho SG, Jung ST, et al. Total ankle arthroplasty following revascularization of avascular necrosis of the talar body: two case reports and literature review. Foot Ankle Int 2008;29(8):852–8.
34. Devalia KL, Ramaskandhan J, Muthumayandi K, et al. Early results of a novel technique: hindfoot fusion in talus osteonecrosis prior to ankle arthroplasty: a case series. Foot (Edinb) 2015;25(4):200–5.
35. Hsu AR, Ellington JK. Patient-specific 3-dimensional printed titanium truss cage with tibiotalocalcaneal arthrodesis for salvage of persistent distal tibia nonunion. Foot Ankle Spec 2015;8(6):483–9.
36. Cohen MM, Kazak M. Tibiocalcaneal arthrodesis with a porous tantalum spacer and locked intramedullary nail for post-traumatic global avascular necrosis of the talus. J Foot Ankle Surg 2015;54(6):1172–7.
37. Palmanovich E, Brin YS, Ben David D, et al. Use of a spinal cage for creating stable constructs in ankle and subtalar fusion. J Foot Ankle Surg 2015;54(2):254–7.
38. Leduc S, Clare MP, Laflamme GY, et al. Posttraumatic avascular necrosis of the talus. Foot Ankle Clin 2008;13(4):753–65.
39. Devries JG, Philbin TM, Hyer CF. Retrograde intramedullary nail arthrodesis for avascular necrosis of the talus. Foot Ankle Int 2010;31(11):965–72.
40. Urquhart MW, Mont MA, Michelson JD, et al. Osteonecrosis of the talus: treatment by hindfoot fusion. Foot Ankle Int 1996;17(5):275–82.
41. Huang YC, Harbst K, Kotajarvi B, et al. Effects of ankle-foot orthoses on ankle and foot kinematics in patients with subtalar osteoarthritis. Arch Phys Med Rehabil 2006;87(8):1131–6.
42. Patzkowski JC, Blanck RV, Owens JG, et al. Comparative effect of orthosis design on functional performance. J Bone Joint Surg Am 2012;94(6):507–15.
43. Highsmith MJ, Nelson LM, Carbone NT, et al. Outcomes associated with the intrepid dynamic exoskeletal orthosis (IDEO): a systematic review of the literature. Mil Med 2016;181(S4):69–76.
44. Perlman MH, Thordarson DB. Ankle fusion in a high risk population: an assessment of nonunion risk factors. Foot Ankle Int 1999;20(8):491–6.
45. De Vries JG, Berlet GC, Hyer CF. Union rate of tibiotalocalcaneal nails with internal or external bone stimulation. Foot Ankle Int 2012;33(11):969–78.
46. Lin SS, Yeranosian MG. The role of orthobiologics in fracture healing and arthrodesis. Foot Ankle Clin 2016;21(4):727–37.
47. Guerkov HH, Lohmann CH, Liu Y, et al. Pulsed electromagnetic fields increase growth factor release by nonunion cells. Clin Orthop Relat Res 2001;(384): 265–79.
48. Saltzman C, Lightfoot A, Amendola A. PEMF as treatment for delayed healing of foot and ankle arthrodesis. Foot Ankle Int 2004;25(11):771–3.
49. Mayr E, Frankel V, Ruter A. Ultrasound–an alternative healing method for nonunions? Arch Orthop Trauma Surg 2000;120(1–2):1–8.

50. Jones CP, Coughlin MJ, Shurnas PS. Prospective CT scan evaluation of hindfoot nonunions treated with revision surgery and low-intensity ultrasound stimulation. Foot Ankle Int 2006;27(4):229–35.
51. Donley BG, Ward DM. Implantable electrical stimulation in high-risk hindfoot fusions. Foot Ankle Int 2002;23(1):13–8.
52. Hockenbury RT, Gruttadauria M, McKinney I. Use of implantable bone growth stimulation in Charcot ankle arthrodesis. Foot Ankle Int 2007;28(9):971–6.
53. Midis N, Conti SF. Revision ankle arthrodesis. Foot Ankle Int 2002;23(3):243–7.
54. Khoury NJ, el-Khoury GY, Saltzman CL, et al. Intraarticular foot and ankle injections to identify source of pain before arthrodesis. AJR Am J Roentgenol 1996; 167(3):669–73.

Tibiotalocalcaneal Arthrodesis for Severe Talar Avascular Necrosis

James R. Lachman, MD, Samuel B. Adams, MD*

KEYWORDS

- Avascular necrosis of the talus • Talar collapse • Tibiotalocalcaneal arthrodesis
- Allograft bone block • 3-D printed cage • 3-D printed truss

KEY POINTS

- Severe talar avascular necrosis is a debilitating problem that, after debridement of dead bone in the operating room, results in large bone voids and presents difficult challenges for the foot and ankle surgeon.
- Patient expectations must be set to achieve realistic goals, including improvements in pain as well as a stable, plantigrade foot.
- Management of bone loss includes block allografts like fresh frozen femoral heads, fresh whole talus allografts, and 3-dimensional printed cages.
- The use of orthobiologics is commonly done to improve healing milieu during arthrodesis. More evidence is needed to support this practice.

INTRODUCTION

The treatment options for avascular necrosis (AVN) of the talus depend on the extent of the disease and whether the adjacent joints are involved.[1–5] Severe AVN of the talus poses a unique challenge to the foot and ankle surgeon. Advanced or severe AVN of the talus indicates significant bone loss or collapse of large portions of the talus. This process can result in structural collapse of the hindfoot, poor function, and pain. The task to replace or span large bone voids, maintain "neutral alignment" (the foot is at a 90° angle to the long axis of the tibia, in neutral or slight external rotation, with 5°–7° of hindfoot valgus), and provide the patient a pain-free or minimally painful plantigrade foot is in the hands of the operating surgeon. These goals can be achieved with careful preoperative planning and fundamental surgical technique, as well as creativity to solve complex, rare problems.

Disclosure: Dr Lachman has nothing to disclose. Dr Adams is a paid consultant for Stryker, Extremity Medical, Orthofix, Medshape.
Department of Orthopaedic Surgery, Duke University, 4709 Creekstone Drive, Durham, NC 27703, USA
* Corresponding author.
E-mail address: Samuel.adams@duke.edu

Foot Ankle Clin N Am 24 (2019) 143–161
https://doi.org/10.1016/j.fcl.2018.11.002

foot.theclinics.com

Appropriate preoperative evaluation includes a comprehensive patient medical history, nutrition and metabolic laboratory values, physical examination, and assessment of hindfoot alignment and standard radiographs (**Fig. 1**), as well as advanced imaging. Laboratory values including vitamin D and calcium, albumin and prealbumin, and a complete metabolic panel can offer insight into whether a patient is even a candidate for surgery and if they have the healing potential as a host to undergo these complicated procedures.[6]

MRI demonstrates the extent of necrosis and can elucidate the areas of bony edema. Low signal intensity of T1-weighted images occurs secondary to adipocyte death, whereas high or mixed signal intensity on T2-weighted images occur owing to increased bony edema (**Fig. 2**).[7] MRI combined with a computed tomography (CT) scan provides 2 components necessary to evaluate bony necrosis.[8] CT imaging can provide a better 3-dimensional (3-D) understanding of collapse and bone loss as well as a complete picture of the bony architecture and alignment after collapse (**Fig. 3**).

Standard treatments for severe talar AVN include arthrodesis with or without bone grafting. This technique has been the most reported that has been used to manage this condition in the orthopedic literature.[9–13] Structural block intercalary bone grafting (**Fig. 4**) has become common practice to fight the complication of limb shortening so common after TTC arthrodesis as well as after talar

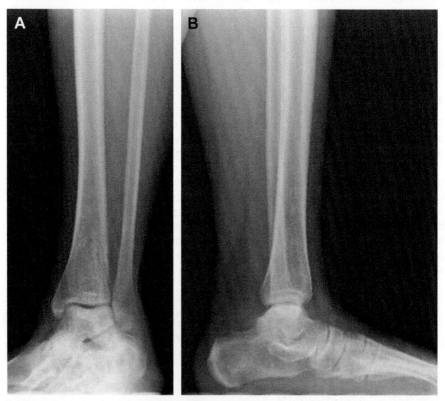

Fig. 1. Anteroposterior (*A*) and lateral (*B*) radiographs demonstrating sclerotic changes in talar body and dome with minimal collapse.

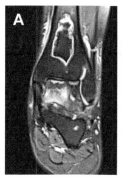
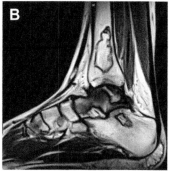
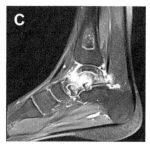

Fig. 2. Coronal (*A*) and sagittal (*B, C*) MRI sequences demonstrating edema and trabecular changes in the talar dome and body.

AVN.[10,12,14,15] With the advent of 3-D printed orthopedic implants, the opportunity to design both custom and noncustom cages or trusses has provided another option to manage this complicated problem. These technological advances add another tool to the armamentarium of the treating surgeon.

This article reviews the treatment of severe AVN of the talus with tibiotalocalcaneal (TTC) arthrodesis. It includes a literature review of the historical techniques used to manage this complicated problem as well as a contemporary review of new techniques developed to avoid pitfalls and problems with the established surgeries. Many studies are available in the literature, which review the results after treating this complex problem. Most are small case series. There are very few large-scale studies and prospective studies are even more rare. The use of 3-D printed titanium trusses has only been used since 2014, so the outcomes data presented, although promising, are only short term. As more and more of these procedures are done, a better understanding of successful techniques and studies including patient reported outcomes will naturally follow.

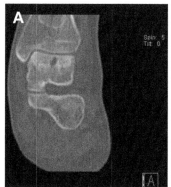
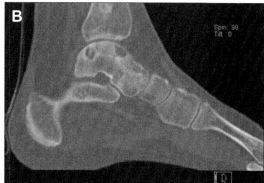

Fig. 3. Coronal (*A*) and sagittal (*B*) computed tomography cuts demonstrating subchondral sclerosis and cyst formation as well as avascular changes to the trabeculae in the talar body and dome.

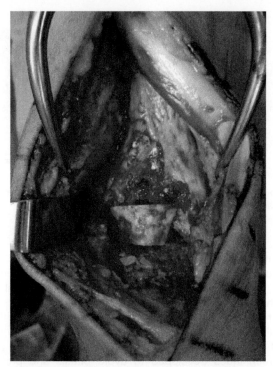

Fig. 4. Structural intercalary allograft from the calcar portion of a femoral head allograft placed into the void created after debridement of necrotic bone in situations of avascular necrosis.

HISTORY

The talus is at risk for vascular insult owing to the nature of its tenuous blood supply.[16,17] Causes of AVN include trauma, hypercortisolism, corticosteroid use, human immunodeficiency virus infection, renal transplantation, alcoholism or pancreatitis, irradiation, multiple sclerosis, collagen vascular disorders, or idiopathic causes.[1–4,18–21] The processes involved in each of these causative conditions varies but the end-organ effect is compromise of the microvasculature and macrovasculature in bone.

Most talar neck fractures result in some degree of talar AVN.[22,23] Many patients will only have minor symptoms and, in cases of minimal AVN, may go on to asymptomatic healing. Some patients may be asymptomatic until sequelae from this process occurs. These sequelae include talar collapse and arthritis of the ankle, subtalar joint, or both; some may progress to an equinovarus deformity of the foot.[24] Controversial treatment considerations for early talar AVN include weightbearing versus nonweightbearing, immobilization versus early range of motion, and conservative versus surgical treatments. When the talar AVN is severe and talar collapse has ensued, management is less controversial.

Severe AVN leads to structural changes in the architecture of the talus as well as compromise of hindfoot alignment. In addition to the subtalar joint, these deformities often involve the tibiotalar joint. Conservative treatment for late-stage talar AVN is rarely successful and has been discussed in this issue. We focus on available surgical techniques for this challenging condition.

SURGICAL TREATMENT OF SEVERE TALAR AVASCULAR NECROSIS

Many techniques have been described to manage the many issues associated with severe talar AVN, including gradual correction with external fixators, osteotomies, and allograft bone blocks shaped to correct the deformity.[3,9–13] Skin contractures as well as scars from previous injuries or surgeries must be considered when determining the most appropriate approach. We present a discussion of fixation methods, void-filling options, and biologic adjuncts currently available, followed by case example illustrations.

FIXATION METHODS

The literature on arthrodesis using an external fixator is limited (**Fig. 5**). Dennison and colleagues[25] reported on 6 cases of talar AVN treated with talectomy and Ilizarov ringed-external fixator arthrodesis. Five of the 6 patients reported good results and all 6 patients went on to union. In a similar case series of arthrodesis secondary to talar AVN, Kitaoka and Patzer[26] reported on 16 cases of tibiotalar calcaneal arthrodesis. In this series, external fixator (12/16), staples (3/16), and no hardware (1/16) were used and these investigators reported a nonunion rate of 19%. Rochman and colleagues[27] reported on their experience with TTC arthrodesis using the Ilizarov technique in 11 patients. Nine of the 11 patients had successful fusions and another fused successfully after revision.

Plates and screws in many combinations have been studied often. Urquhart and colleagues[11] treated 11 patients with arthrodesis using plates and screws after talar AVN. The authors reported 9 excellent results and 2 infected nonunions, one of which required below knee amputation. Fan and colleagues[28] reported on their experience with TTC arthrodesis using a transfibular approach and locked plating. Of the 12 cases included in the study, 3 patients suffered from talar AVN. All 3 patients went

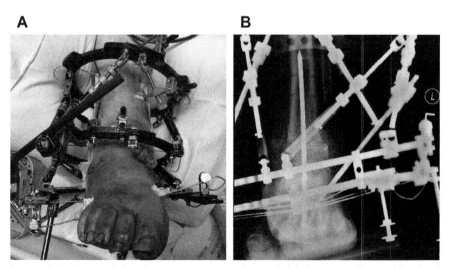

Fig. 5. Clinical image (A) and anteroposterior radiograph (B) demonstrating a tibiotalocal-caneal arthrodesis using ringed external fixation and block allograft.

on to successful arthrodesis (average time to arthrodesis of 2.8 months) and all had significant improvement in American Orthopaedic Foot and Ankle Society hindfoot scores.

TTC arthrodesis using an intramedullary nail has been widely reported. Tenenbaum and colleagues[29] reported on 14 limbs that underwent TTC arthrodesis for talar AVN using retrograde intramedullary nailing. All patients went on to union and Short Form-36, American Orthopaedic Foot and Ankle Society hindfoot, and visual analogue scale scores improved across the cohort. Jeng and colleagues[10] reported on 33 cases of TTC arthrodesis using a retrograde intramedullary nail. Six of these patients underwent this procedure owing to talar AVN. Three went on to nonunion requiring revision surgery in this cohort. DeVries and colleagues[9] shared their experience with TTC arthrodesis using a retrograde intramedullary nail for treatment of talar AVN in 14 patients. Twelve patients went on to union and 2 patients went on to stable pseudarthrosis. Four patients developed minor postoperative complications and no patient in the cohort required major revision surgery. In all of these studies cited, a bone graft was used to supplement the arthrodesis. Freeze-dried or fresh frozen bulk femoral head allografts were used most often .

FILLING THE VOID

Historically, restoration of limb length, structural substitution in cases of large bony voids, and deformity correction have all been addressed with intercalary structural autograft or allograft. Many small case series are available in the literature with arthrodesis rates ranging from 50% to 93%.[3,9–14,21,25–30] Structural bone grafts require healing through the interfaces between the graft and the native bone and risks future collapse if this incorporation is not successful. Over time, even with successful fusion, some collapse is common.

Bulk Femoral Head Allograft

Jeng and colleagues[10] reported on the results of 32 patients who underwent TTC arthrodesis using bulk femoral head allograft to fill large bony voids. The defects were the result of talar AVN, failed total ankle replacement, trauma, osteomyelitis, Charcot foot, or failed reconstructive surgery. Sixteen patients healed their fusion for an overall success rate of 50%. Diabetes mellitus was listed as a predictive factor for failure. All 9 patients with diabetes developed a nonunion. In this series, 19% of patients went on to a below-knee amputation.

Bussewitz and colleagues[30] published a series of 25 patients who underwent femoral head allograft and TTC intramedullary nail for complex hindfoot and ankle reconstruction. Twelve patients went on to successful fusion, 21 patients had a braceable limb, and 4 patients required major amputation.[30]

Tenenbaum and colleagues[29] published a more recent series following 10 patients who underwent TTC arthrodesis and bone grafting secondary to AVN of the talus. The authors report a 100% union rate. Patient-reported outcomes included American Orthopedic Foot and Ankle Society Score, visual analogue scale, and Short Form-36. All outcomes measures showed significant improvement after surgery. There were 6 complications in this series, the most common being painful hardware requiring removal in 4 patients.

Titanium Cages

Recently, 3-D printing has become available for use in medical implants. Space-occupying cages or trusses provide an opportunity to avoid collapse or nonunion secondary to poor incorporation of block allograft bone. These cages can be packed with allograft or autograft bone and can fit into prepared spaces, much like bulk femoral head allografts. This concept, although new to foot and ankle surgery, has been used in other areas of orthopedics with repeated success. Spine surgeons have used autologous bone in combination with titanium cages for arthrodesis in areas with vertebral defects for years with arthrodesis rates ranging from 76.0% to 97.7%.[31–33] Implant cost has been discussed and, ignoring the cost of donor allograft bone blocks, the surgical time saved fashioning a bone graft to fit the void offsets this cost.[32]

Careful preoperative planning is essential to identify patients who are good candidates for this procedure. A CT scan of the affected side establishes the bone loss in the talus owing to AVN. A CT scan of the contralateral limb (assuming pathology is not bilateral) provides the 3-D printing company a template for baseline dimensions and height restoration. The surgeon, working closely with the design team, can correct deformity, bone loss, and provide limb length restoration by creating an implant that addresses all of these problems.

As indicated elsewhere in this issue, the literature on 3-D printed titanium truss augmented arthrodesis in the foot and ankle is sparse. Early results using titanium cages (not 3-D printed) were less than promising. Carlsson[34] reported on the use of a titanium mesh cage in ankle arthrodesis after failed ankle replacement in 3 patients. The cages were placed into the void and none of the ankles went on to union. All 3 patients required revision surgery. Bullens and colleagues[35] published a case series with 2 patients who underwent TTC arthrodesis with retrograde intramedullary nail using and intercalary mesh cage to fill a large bone void. One of the patients went on to nonunion by 6 months and the other had significant collapse and hardware failure although, clinically had improved.

More recently, Preston and colleagues[36] published a case report on a patient treated with TTC arthrodesis after failed total ankle arthroplasty using 3-D printed titanium truss, which accommodated a retrograde intramedullary nail. By 16 weeks, the patient progressed to full weightbearing and returned to activities of daily living in a sneaker with a gauntlet ankle brace. Another case report by Hsu and Ellington[37] documented the use of a custom 3-D printed truss for hindfoot arthrodesis after distal tibia nonunion using a retrograde intramedullary nail. At the patient's most recent follow-up, they were ambulating without assistive device for the first time in 2 years since the index injury. Mulhern and colleagues[38] reported on a patient whom had a large bone void secondary to infected TAA and talar component subsidence. A titanium truss was inserted and at the most recent follow-up, the patient was pain free and weightbearing with a CT scan confirming bony consolidation through the cage. These case studies report on the use of 3-D printed implants used after failed total ankle replacement or trauma.

In the largest study to date looking at the results of patient-specific 3-D–printed titanium cage implants used in 15 patients, Dekker and colleagues[39] found radiographic fusion in 13 of 15 using CT scans. The cages were used in scenarios of severe bone loss, deformity correction, and/or arthrodesis procedures. The study included patient-reported outcomes scores (visual analogue scale, the Foot and Ankle Ability Measure Activities of Daily Living score, and the American Orthopedic Foot and Ankle Score), which all demonstrates significant improvements postoperatively. In the 2 failures, one patient failed owing to infection and the other failed owing to nonunion.

BIOLOGIC ADDITIVES

Whether using bulk autograft or allograft bone or 3-D printed cages or trusses packed with bone, establishing a milieu conducive to healing is essential. The market for ortho-biologics has exploded over the past decade and the literature on optimal conditions for bone healing, although currently limited, is promising. To optimize bone healing potential, a construct that has mechanical stability and provides an environment that is osteoconductive, osteoinductive, and angiogenic is preferred. Proper joint preparation, rigid fixation, careful soft tissue management, and supplementation with ortho-biologics can provide the desired environment. A thorough review of contemporary orthobiologics is beyond the scope of this article.

These authors prefer to pack the titanium truss with either allograft or autograft cancellous bone soaked in recombinant human platelet-derived growth factor B homodimer (AUGMENT, Wright Medical, Memphis, TN), allograft recombinant human bone morphogenic protein, or allograft adult mesenchymal stem cells or autograft bone marrow aspirate concentrate (**Figs. 6** and **7**).

CASE EXAMPLE 1 (BLOCK ALLOGRAFT)
History

A 63-year-old woman with a 5-year history of pain in the midfoot and sinus tarsi presented for treatment. She underwent a midfoot and subtalar arthrodesis 3 years ago, which alleviated her pain for approximately 18 months postoperatively. One year previously, she began having debilitating pain in her ankle and hindfoot, which progressed until she was unable to bear weight. Initial weightbearing radiographs demonstrated near complete collapse of the talus and hindfoot varus deformity with hardware passing through the sinus tarsi (**Fig. 8**). Her talar AVN was likely iatrogenic secondary to the index surgery. She was scheduled for hardware removal, debridement of necrotic bone, and fresh talar allograft with TTC arthrodesis using an intramedullary nail.

Surgical Technique

The patient was placed supine on the operating table and a standard direct anterior approach to the ankle was used to expose the tibiotalar and talonavicular joints. After thorough debridement of necrotic bone, it was clear that the entire talus was not viable

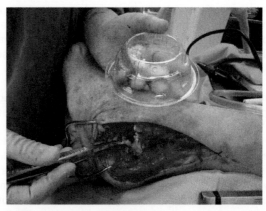

Fig. 6. Use of MAP3 (RTI surgical Inc. Alachua, FL) in the prepared surface before grafting.

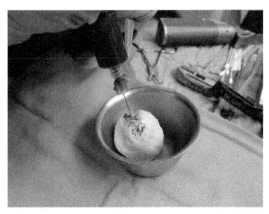

Fig. 7. Injecting iliac crest bone marrow aspirate concentrate into the femoral head allograft in preparation for implantation.

and needed to be removed. The surfaces of the calcaneus and tibia were prepared by removing all sclerotic subchondral bone and fenestrating the surfaces with a 2.5-mm drill and chisels. A fresh allograft whole talus was prepared by removing all cartilage and this block graft was placed in the void created by debridement of the necrotic talus. Allograft recombinant human bone morphogenic protein as well as allograft adult mesenchymal stem cells were used to supplement the fusion sites. The allograft talus was then secured with guidewires, which could accommodate headless, cannulated compression screws (**Fig. 9**).

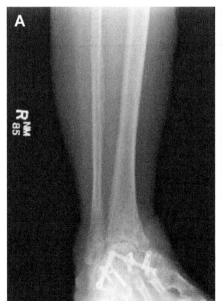
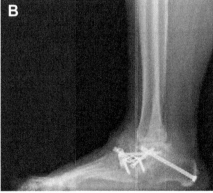

Fig. 8. Anteroposterior (*A*) and lateral (*B*) radiographs of patient described in case example 1. Previous hardware traversing the sinus tarsi is evident.

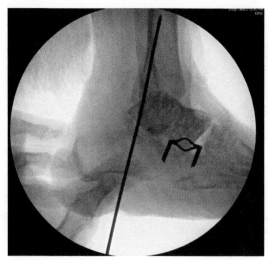

Fig. 9. Intraoperative fluoroscopic lateral radiograph demonstrating fresh frozen whole talar allograft held in place with a guidewire for a cannulated screw.

A standard retrograde intramedullary TTC nail was placed through the calcaneus, allograft talus and tibia, being sure to maintain the desired neutral alignment (**Fig. 10**). The nail was then secured in compression with proximal and distal interlocking screws. Supplemental fixation was added in the talonavicular joint as well as the TTC construct with cannulated compression screws. Finally, an anterior plate was placed for additional structural support (**Fig. 11**).

Postoperative Management

Preoperative laboratory tests demonstrated vitamin D deficiency, so the patient was placed on oral vitamin D and calcium supplementation for the duration of

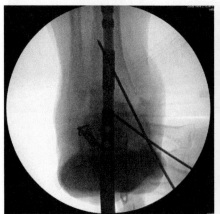
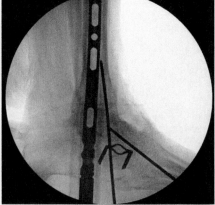

Fig. 10. Intraoperative fluoroscopic radiographs demonstrating nail position through the whole talar allograft along with supplementary fixation.

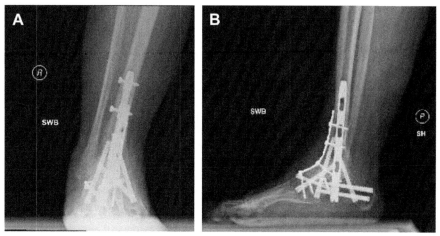

Fig. 11. Anteroposterior (*A*) and lateral (*B*) radiographs taken at 3 months postoperatively demonstrating the maintenance of alignment and some early bony consolidation at arthrodesis sites.

the treatment. The patient was kept nonweightbearing in a cast for 3 months and then placed into a pneumatic walking boot to begin gradual weightbearing. Repeat CT scans at 6 months demonstrated bony consolidation at all 3 arthrodesis sites.

CASE EXAMPLE 2 (BULK ALLOGRAFT FEMORAL HEAD)
History

A 54-year-old man with a history of a right talus fracture treated nonoperatively in a cast at an outside hospital now presents 4 years later complaining of ankle and hind-foot pain. Radiographs revealed AVN of the talus with collapse of the talar body (**Fig. 12**). He failed nonoperative treatment in an Arizona brace and was indicated for bulk femoral head allograft with retrograde intramedullary nail TTC arthrodesis. The patient was an active smoker in the months before presentation in the clinic and was counseled that surgery would not be possible until the patient was nicotine free for at least 6 weeks preoperatively. After negative nicotine screening the patient underwent the procedure.

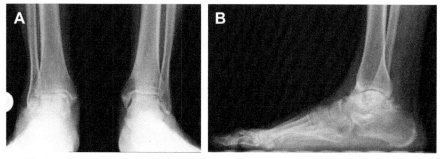

Fig. 12. Anteroposterior (*A*) and lateral (*B*) radiographs corresponding to case example 2 showing subchondral sclerosis and early collapse of the talar dome and body.

Surgical Technique

The patient was placed prone on the operating table and a standard direct posterior approach to the ankle splitting the Achilles tendon was used to expose the collapsed, necrotic talar body and dome. After thorough debridement of avascular bone, it was evident that there was a large defect (**Fig. 13**). Height was restored using a lamina spreader and the femoral head allograft was sized. Using the smallest available acetabular reamer (38 mm), the cavity was prepared by removing subchondral sclerotic bone and exposing bleeding surfaces (**Fig. 14**). A bulk femoral head allograft was prepared by removing all cartilage and this block graft was placed in the void created by the reaming (**Figs. 15** and **16**). Allograft recombinant human bone morphogenic protein as well as allograft adult mesenchymal stem cells were used to supplement the fusion sites. The allograft femoral head was then secured with guidewires, which could accommodate headless, cannulated compression screws if possible (**Fig. 17**).

A standard retrograde intramedullary TTC nail was placed through the calcaneus, allograft femoral head, and tibia, being sure to maintain the desired neutral alignment. The nail was then secured in compression with proximal and distal interlocking screws (**Fig. 18**).

Postoperative Management

Continued antismoking counseling was done at each postoperative visit. Per protocol, the patient was kept nonweightbearing in a cast for 3 months and then placed into a pneumatic walking boot to begin gradual weightbearing. Radiographic fusion was noticed at the patient's 6-month postoperative visit.

CASE EXAMPLE 3 (3-DIMENSIONAL PRINTED TITANIUM TRUSS/CAGE)
History

A 29-year-old woman with a history of ulcerative colitis and chronic steroid use presented with complaints of chronic left ankle pain that was refractory to nonoperative treatments. She was diagnosed with AVN of the talar body with early collapse. She had previously undergone core decompression at an outside hospital through an anterior approach, which was unsuccessful. Radiographs, MRI, and CT scans are shown

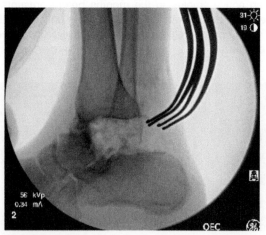

Fig. 13. Intraoperative lateral radiograph demonstrating a large void after necrotic bone was debrided.

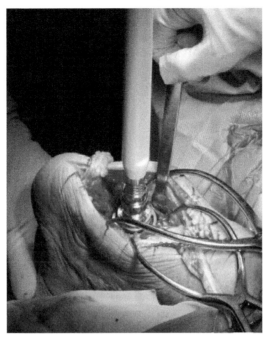

Fig. 14. Intraoperative clinical photograph demonstrating the use of the acetabular reamer to prepare the bony surfaces to accept the femoral head allograft.

in **Figs. 1–7**. She was indicated for a retrograde TTC arthrodesis using a patient-specific 3-D–printed titanium truss.

Surgical Technique

The 3-D printing orthopedic implant company used for this case requires a minimum of 3 weeks' notice to engineer and manufacture the implant. CT scans of both ankles are

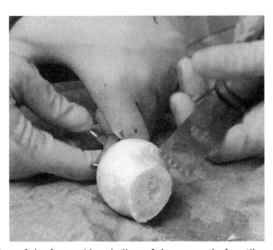

Fig. 15. Preparation of the femoral head allograft by removal of cartilage and subchondral bone.

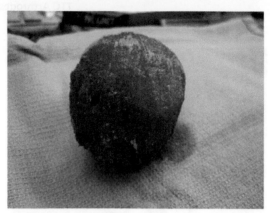

Fig. 16. The prepared femoral head allograft soaked in bone marrow aspirate concentrate.

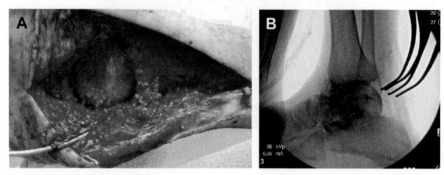

Fig. 17. Clinical photograph (A) and Intraoperative fluoroscopic lateral (B) demonstrating the prepared femoral head allograft in position.

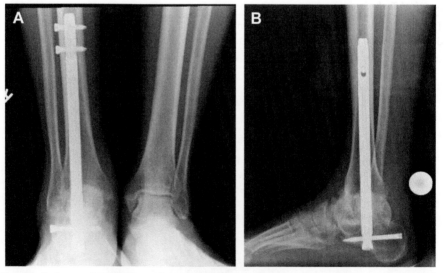

Fig. 18. Anteroposterior (A) and lateral (B) radiographs taken at 6 months postoperatively showing a tibiotalocalcaneal arthrodesis nail in place and consolidation of the arthrodesis sites between the tibia and femoral head allograft as well as the calcaneus and femoral head allograft.

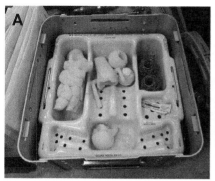
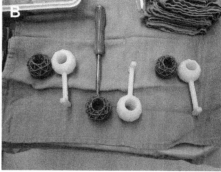

Fig. 19. Patient-specific 3-dimensional printed truss and trials in the tray (*A*) and then laid out on the back table in the operating room (*B*).

required to engineer the implant in the most accurate way. The company used in this case prints 4 total implants that included a central canal to accommodate an IM nail; multiple sizes can be printed including volumetrically larger and smaller implants with associated trials (**Fig. 19**).

A direct posterior approach was used in the prone position. Once the posterior ankle and subtalar joints were visualized, all necrotic bone was removed. Using the acetabular reamers and fluoroscopy, the bed was reamed to the size appropriate to fit the implant. Trials with handles attached are printed as well, which match the full-sized implants in all the available sizes (**Fig. 20**). Through trialing, the appropriate size is determined and then placed into the prepared void, ensuring the canal for the intramedullary nail is in the appropriate orientation. Some maneuvering is required to pass the sequential reamers for the nail through the trial so as not to compromise the truss (**Fig. 21**).

A standard retrograde intramedullary TTC nail was placed through the calcaneus, 3-D printed titanium truss, and tibia, being sure to maintain the desired neutral alignment. The cage was filled with autograft bone obtained from the acetabular reamings and allograft adult mesenchymal stem cells (**Figs. 22** and **23**).

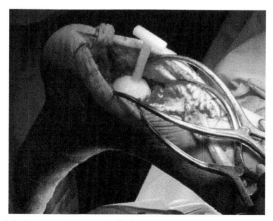

Fig. 20. Trialing with the 2 options provided to ensure the appropriate fit.

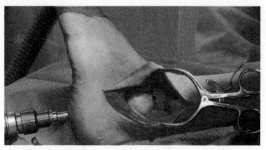

Fig. 21. Reaming through the trial (viewed from a lateral approach in a different patient) to avoid compromise of the 3-dimensional printed titanium implant.

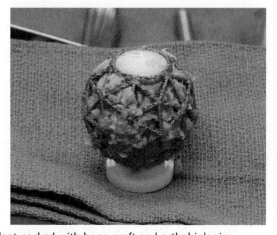

Fig. 22. The implant packed with bone graft and orthobiologics.

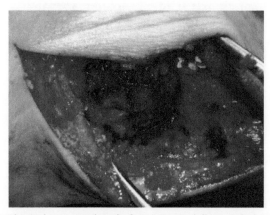

Fig. 23. Prepared spherical truss in place before intramedullary nail placement.

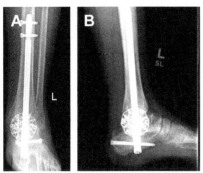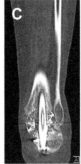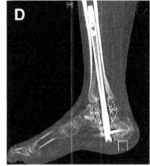

Fig. 24. Anteroposterior (*A*) and lateral (*B*) radiographs, and coronal (*C*) and sagittal (*D*) computed tomography scans at 6 months postoperatively demonstrating a spherical cage in place with a retrograde intramedullary nail passing through it.

Postoperative Management

The patient was treated nonweightbearing in a cast for 3 months and then placed into a pneumatic walking boot to begin gradual weightbearing. A CT scan at 6 months demonstrated incorporation and bony ingrowth of the truss at both the tibial and calcaneal interfaces (**Fig. 24**).

SUMMARY

Severe talar AVN results from many different etiologies resulting in bone loss and hindfoot deformity requiring surgical intervention to maintain a plantigrade foot. Tibiotalar calcaneal arthrodesis is a salvage procedure after severe talar AVN. Large bone voids spanning 2 or 3 articulations can present significant challenges to the treating surgeon.

Modest successes have been reported with structural block allograft TTC arthrodesis using either plate and screws, intramedullary nail fixation or a combination of the two. The advent of 3-D printed titanium trusses has given surgeons another option for filling voids creates by bone loss and providing structural support to prevent collapse. Although these options expand the armamentarium, treating surgeons must still adhere to principles of arthrodesis including stable constructs, thorough joint surface preparation, and correction of deformity.

REFERENCES

1. Chiodo CP, Herbst SA. Osteonecrosis of the talus. Foot Ankle Clin 2004;9: 745–55, vi.
2. Delanois RE, Mont MA, Yoon TR, et al. Atraumatic osteonecrosis of the talus. J Bone Joint Surg Am 1998;80:529–36.
3. Horst F, Gilbert BJ, Nunley JA. Avascular necrosis of the talus: current treatment options. Foot Ankle Clin 2004;9:757–73.
4. Adelaar RS, Madrian JR. Avascular necrosis of the talus. Orthop Clin North Am 2004;35:383–95.
5. Mont MA, Schon LC, Hungerford MW, et al. Avascular necrosis of the talus treated by core decompression. J Bone Joint Surg Br 1996;78:827–30.
6. Gorter EA, Hamdy NA, Appelman-Dijkstra NM, et al. The role of vitamin D in human fracture healing: a systematic review of the literature. Bone 2014;64:288–97.

7. Chen H, Liu W, Deng L, et al. The prognostic value of the Hawkins sign and diagnostic value to MRI after talar neck fractures. Foot Ankle Int 2014;35(12):1255–61.

8. Henderson RC. Posttraumatic necrosis of the talus: the Hawkins sign versus magnetic resonance imaging. J Orthop Trauma 1991;5:96–9.

9. DeVries JG, Philbin TM, Hyer CF. Retrograde intramedullary nail arthrodesis for avascular necrosis of the talus. Foot Ankle Int 2010;31(11):965–72.

10. Jeng CL, Campbell JT, Tang EY, et al. Tibiotalocalcaneal arthrodesis with bulk femoral head allograft for salvage of large defects in the ankle. Foot Ankle Int 2013;34(9):1256–66.

11. Urquhart MW, Mont MA, Michelson JD, et al. Osteonecrosis of the talus: treatment by hindfoot fusion. Foot Ankle Int 1996;17(5):275–82.

12. Clowers BE, Myerson MS. A novel surgical technique for the management of massive osseous defects in the hindfoot with bulk allograft. Foot Ankle Clin 2011;16:181–9.

13. Royer C, Brodsky JW. Arthrodesis techniques for avascular necrosis of the talus. Tech Foot Ankle Surg 2002;l(l):50–9.

14. Berkowitz MJ, Clare MP, Walling AK, et al. Salvage of failed total ankle arthroplasty with fusion using structural allograft and internal fixation. Foot Ankle Int 2011;32:S493–502.

15. Myerson MS, Neufeld SK, Uribe J. Fresh-frozen structural allografts in the foot and ankle. J Bone Joint Surg Am 2005;87:113–20.

16. Kelly PJ, Sullivan CR. Blood supply of the talus. Clin Orthop 1963;30:37–44.

17. Mulfinger GL, Trueta J. The blood supply of the talus. J Bone Joint Surg 1970; 52B:160–7.

18. Baron M, Paltiel H, Lander P. Aseptic necrosis of the talus and calcaneal insufficiency fractures in a patient with pancreatitis, subcutaneous fat necrosis, and arthritis. Arthritis Rheum 1984;27:1309–13.

19. Adleberg JS, Smith GH. Corticosteroid-induced avascular necrosis of the talus. J Foot Surg 1991;30:66–9.

20. Kemnitz S, Moens P, Peerlinck K, et al. Avascular necrosis of the talus in children with haemophilia. J Pediatr Orthop B 2002;11:73–8.

21. Kolker D, Wilson MG. Tibiocalcaneal arthrodesis after total talectomy for treatment of osteomyelitis of the talus. Foot Ankle Int 2004;25:861–5.

22. Canale ST, Kelly FB Jr. Fractures of the neck of the talus. Long-term evaluation of seventy-one cases. J Bone Joint Surg Am 1978;60:143–56.

23. Leduc S, Clare MP, Laflamme GY, et al. Posttraumatic avascular necrosis of the talus. Foot Ankle Clin 2008;13:753–65.

24. Hawkins LG. Fractures of the neck of the talus. J Bone Joint Surg Am 1970;52: 991–1002.

25. Dennison MG, Pool RD, Simonis RB, et al. Tibiocalcaneal fusion for avascular necrosis of the talus. J Bone Joint Surg Br 2001;83:199–203.

26. Kitaoka HB, Patzer GL. Arthrodesis for the treatment of arthrosis of the ankle and osteonecrosis of the talus. J Bone Joint Surg Am 1998;80:370–9.

27. Rochman R, Jackson Hutson J, Alade O. Tibiocalcaneal arthrodesis using the Ilizarov technique in the presence of bone loss and infection of the talus. Foot Ankle Int 2008;29:1001–8.

28. Fan J, Zhang X, Luo Y, et al. Tibiotalocalcaneal arthrodesis with reverse PHILOS plate and medial cannulated screws with lateral approach. BMC Musculoskelet Disord 2017;18:317.

29. Tenenbaum S, Stockton KG, Bariteau JT, et al. Salvage of avascular necrosis of the talus by combined ankle and hindfoot arthrodesis with structural bone graft. Foot Ankle Int 2015;36(3):282–7.
30. Bussewitz B, DeVries JG, Dejula M, et al. Retrograde intramedullary nail with femoral head allograft for large deficit tibiotalocalcaneal arthrodesis. Foot Ankle Int 2014;35(7):706–11.
31. Callanan TC, Walker B, Grinberg S, et al. Prospective, 88 patient series study of the use of a novel 3-D printed titanium truss system cage in anterior cervical spinal surgery. Spine J 2016;16(10):S360.
32. Wilcox B, Mobbs RJ, Wu A, et al. Systematic review of 3D printing in spinal surgery: the current state of play. J Spine Surg 2017;3(3):433–43.
33. Mobbs RJ, Phan K, Malham G, et al. Lumbar interbody fusion: techniques and comparison of interbody fusion options including PLIF, TLIF, MI-TLIF, OLIF/ATP, LLIF and ALIF. J Spine Surg 2015;1(1):2–18.
34. Carlsson A. Unsuccessful use of titanium mesh cage in ankle arthrodesis: a report on three cases operated on due to failed total ankle replacement. J Foot Ankle Surg 2008;47(4):337–42.
35. Bullens P, de Wall Malefjit M, Louwerens JW. Conversion of failed ankle arthroplasty to an arthrodesis. Technique using an arthrodesis nail and a cage filled with morsellized bone graft. J Foot Ankle Surg 2010;16(2):101–4.
36. Preston NL, Wilson M, Hewitt EA. Salvage arthrodesis of failed total ankle replacement using a custom 3D-printed cage implant: a case report and review of the literature. Proceedings of Singapore Healthcare. Epublished March 7, 2018.
37. Hsu AR, Ellington JK. Patient-specific 3-dimensional printed titanium truss case with tibiotalocalcaneal arthrodesis for salvage of persistent distal tibia nonunion. Foot Ankle Spec 2015;8(6):483–9.
38. Mulhern JL, Protzman NM, White AM, et al. Salvage of failed total ankle replacement using a custom titanium truss. J Foot Ankle Surg 2016;55(4):868–73.
39. Dekker TJ, Steele JR, Federer AE, et al. Use of patient-specific 3D-printed titanium implants for complex foot and ankle limb salvage, deformity correction, and arthrodesis procedures. Foot Ankle Int 2018;39(8):916–21.

An Alumina Ceramic Total Talar Prosthesis for Avascular Necrosis of the Talus

Akira Taniguchi, MD, PhD*, Yasuhito Tanaka, MD, PhD

KEYWORDS

- Aseptic necrosis • Talus • Total talar prosthesis • Alumina ceramic

KEY POINTS

- The talus is surrounded by the tibia, fibula, calcaneus, and navicular, composing some joints in between with these bones.
- Customized alumina ceramic total talar prosthesis is an ideal implant for the replacement due to talar osteonecrosis.
- Preservation of joint function and prevention of leg length discrepancy are important to treat talar osteonecrosis.
- In the authors' experience of 55 ankles in 41 patients with talar osteonecrosis, both subjective and objective scale scores improved after the replacement with customized alumina ceramic total talar prosthesis.

INTRODUCTION

The talus is surrounded by the tibia, fibula, calcaneus, and navicular, and approximately 70% of its surface is covered with articular cartilage. The medial segment of the talus is supplied by the tarsal tunnel artery, branched by the posterior tibial artery. The head and neck of the talus are mainly supplied by the tarsal tunnel and anterior tibial arteries.[1,2] However, avascular necrosis tends to occur in the talus because of poor blood supply from the periosteum.

The causes of talar osteonecrosis are trauma,[3,4] excessive steroid use,[5] alcohol,[6] systemic lupus erythematosus,[6] pancreatitis,[7] hemophilia,[8,9] and severe acute respiratory syndrome.[10] The frequency of talar osteonecrosis associated with talar fracture has been reported to be approximately 10%, 40%, and 90% in Hawkins types 1, 2, and 3,[11] respectively. More recently, talar osteonecrosis frequency decreased to 64%, even in type 3, because of the improved surgical

Disclosure Statement: The authors have nothing to disclose.
Department of Orthopaedic Surgery, Nara Medical University, 840 Shijyo-cho, Kashihara, Nara 631-8522, Japan
* Corresponding author.
E-mail address: a-tani@naramed-u.ac.jp

Foot Ankle Clin N Am 24 (2019) 163–171
https://doi.org/10.1016/j.fcl.2018.10.004
1083-7515/19/© 2018 Elsevier Inc. All rights reserved.

foot.theclinics.com

techniques and implants.[3] However, the frequency of talar osteonecrosis in patients with talar fracture dislocation is still higher. Steroid use increases the blood level of fat, which induces microcontusions, leading to osteonecrosis.[5] Delanois and colleagues[12] reported that 20 of 24 subjects with traumatic talar osteonecrosis had a history of steroid therapy. However, no evidence supports the correlation.

Blair fusion used to be adapted for this condition because it uses the healthy talar neck.[13,14] Although minimal discrepancy of the lower leg remains after this procedure, hindfoot instability and non union in the fixation site sometimes occurred. In some cases, iliac crest harvest and external fixator may be necessary.

The customized alumina ceramic talar prosthesis was developed in 1994 to compensate for the disadvantages of fusion treatments.[15,16] The first-generation implant was a talar body prosthesis with a bone peg for cement fixation to the talar neck. However, some cases had loosening at the fixation site. In 2004, the second-generation implant was designed as a talar body prosthesis without a bone peg and was expected to perform the bearing function on the talar body. However, talar head rupture occurred in some cases because of higher pressure to the talar head. Therefore, total talar prosthesis was developed in 2005 and has been used since. In this article, diagnosis and treatment of talar osteonecrosis, as well as surgical technique for artificial talus implantation, are discussed.

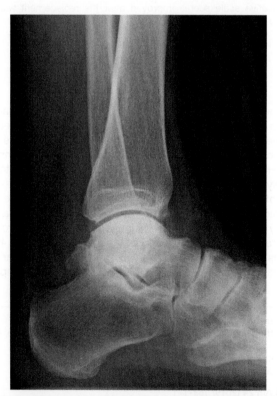

Fig. 1. Radiograph of a 57-year-old man with a vascular necrosis of the talus. Otosclerosis is seen in the body of the talus.

DIAGNOSIS

An etiologic factor of osteonecrosis is that bone ischemia is induced by blood flow disturbance. The cycle of ossification, revascularization, and reabsorption is repeated for the healing system. In early-phase radiography, little difference is seen compared with healthy bone. Next, reabsorption revolves around the necrotic bone, which induces bone atrophy followed by decreased bone stock. In the center of osteonecrosis, sclerotic change appears because of blood flow disruption.

Radiographic staging of osteonecrosis was developed by Ficat and Arlet[17] and was modified for the ankle by Mont and Colleagues[18] Stage 1 is defined as no radiographic findings, stage 2 is defined as cystic lesion and/or sclerotic change in the talus, stage 3 is defined as crescent sign or collapse in the subchondral bone, and stage 4 is defined as joint space narrowing.

In some patients with trauma to the talus, the clear zone can be recognized in the subchondral bone after 6 to 8 weeks of trauma, even in cases with initial sclerotic change, by the restoration of blood flow and that it is free from osteonecrosis (Hawkins sign).

Patients with atraumatic talar osteonecrosis usually consult physicians because of relatively minor ankle pain. Sclerotic change in the talar body would be observed even in cases without severe collapse in the talus (**Fig. 1**). The sagittal and coronal planes of a computed tomography (CT) image reveal sclerotic change in the bony structure of the talus (**Fig. 2**)[19]. Moreover, a 3-dimensional image makes the evaluation of the

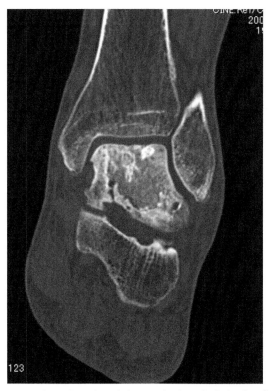

Fig. 2. CT of the same patient. Otosclerosis is seen in the whole body of the talus.

collapse of the talar body and selection of the surgical option possible. In patients treated with artificial talus, CT of the contralateral ankle should be obtained to make a customized implant.

MRI is useful for the detection of early lesions.[19] In the T1-weighted image, the lesion is visualized in the low-density area, reflecting loss of fatty bone marrow. In the T2-weighted image, the lesion is visualized in the high-density and low-density areas, reflecting bone marrow edema in the early and advanced stages, respectively. In the fat-suppressed T2-weighted image, a mixture of high-intensity and low-intensity areas is seen, reflecting bone marrow edema and necrosis, respectively (**Fig. 3**).

Bone scintigraphy has potential diagnostic power to detect the early phase.[20] Although other modalities evaluate only the local tissue, bone scintigraphy targets the whole body, which is an advantage for the diagnosis of atraumatic necrosis. The lesion has a cold area, reflecting the lack of uptake due to necrosis, and a hot area around the cold area reflecting the higher uptake results from reabsorption (cold in hot) (**Fig. 4**).

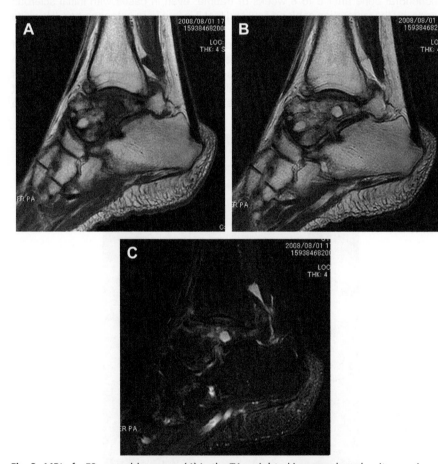

Fig. 3. MRI of a 52-year-old woman. (*A*) In the T1-weighted image, a low-density area is seen in the body of the talus. (*B*) In the T2-weighted image, a high-density area is seen in the body of the talus, and bony cyst is identified in it. (*C*) In fat-suppressed T2-weighted image, a mixture of high-intensity and low-intensity areas is seen, reflecting bone marrow edema and necrosis, respectively.

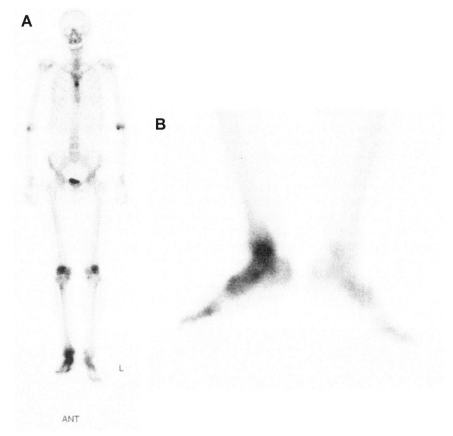

Fig. 4. 99mTc-HMDP bone scintigraphy of a 50-year-old man. (*A*) 99mTc-HMDP (hydroxy-methylene diphosphonate) concentrates to the right talus. (*B*) The lesion has a cold area, re-flecting the lack of uptake due to necrosis, and a hot area around the cold area, reflecting the higher uptake results from reabsorption (cold in hot).

TREATMENT

For patients with stage 1 or 2 without evidence of collapse, dislocation, or degenerative changes in the talus, nonweightbearing using crutches or a knee-bearing orthosis is indicated. Partial weightbearing is allowed after bone resorption is recognized because this indicates the restoration of the blood supply, whereas nonweightbearing may continue long-term in cases without findings of bone resorption.[21] Surgical treatment is considered in patients not responding to conservative therapy.[18] For patients with stage 1 or 2, core decompression technique would be used. Drills of 1.5 mm to 2.0 mm in diameter are inserted into the lesion 5 to 10 times from the posterolateral, lateral, or medial sides, or a drill of 4.0 mm in diameter is inserted 2 to 4 times to reduce the pressure in the lesion. Horst and colleagues[21] reported decreased pain and improved ankle motion in 70% of subjects after this procedure.

For patients with stage 3 and 4, surgical treatment is usually selected, particularly in patients with talar collapse. Tibiocalcaneal fusion connecting the tibia and calcaneus after resecting the collapsed talar body usually results in length discrepancy of the lower legs. Blair fusion connecting the tibia and talar neck with the fibula results in less discrepancy; however, long-term mounting of the external fixator is required to address instability in the fixation site.[13,14] Recently introduced artificial talar prostheses prevent leg length discrepancy, preserve the joint function, and allow early weightbearing.[15,16]

CT of the healthy side of the talus is obtained to make a customized implant. CT images are reconstructed in the pitch of 2 mm in the coronal and sagittal planes. The talar area is identified in each slice, the reconstructed image of the talus is reversed, and the implant is made using this image (**Fig. 5**A–F). The customized ceramic implant is produced in 4 to 5 weeks (**Fig. 5**G); therefore, preventing further collapse of the talus caused by weightbearing is necessary.

Under spinal or general anesthesia, a 10-cm skin incision is made in the anterior ankle. The extensor retinaculum is incised, avoiding damage to the superficial peroneal nerve, and the ankle is exposed between the flexor hallucis longus and tibialis anterior tendons. In addition, the talonavicular joint is exposed in the distal side. After the dissection of the joint capsule and ligaments, the talar neck is cut and the talar head is removed. The talar body is cut 1-cm thick on the coronal plane, dissecting the interosseous talocalcaneal ligament. Removal of the entire bone fragment without retaining small fragments in the surgical site is important. After irrigation of

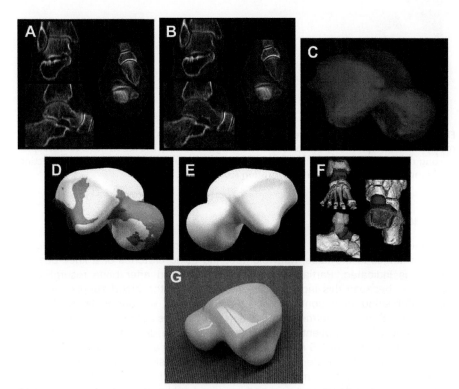

Fig. 5. Creating the customized artificial talus. (*A*) CT scan of the healthy side. (*B*) Distinction of the talus. (*C*) Rending and CAD (Computer Aided Designing) imaging. (*D*) Correction of CAD image. (*E*) Turnover of the image. (*F*) Simulation in the 3-dimensional CT. (*G*) Finished alumina ceramic total talar prosthesis.

the surgical site, the artificial talus is inserted with assistance of foot traction. The ankle, subtalar, and talonavicular joints are ranged to confirm good prosthetic fit. The surgical wound is closed following joint capsule repair (**Fig. 6**). A below-knee walking cast is applied for 3 weeks. Weightbearing is avoided in the first week, partial weightbearing is allowed in the second week, and full weightbearing is allowed in the third week (**Fig. 7**).

In the authors' experience of 55 ankles in 41 patients with talar osteonecrosis, the Japanese Society for Surgery of the Foot Ankle–Hindfoot Scale score improved from 42.2 plus or minus 17.4 to 89.1 plus or minus 8.6. In the subcategory of pain, score improved from 15.0 plus or minus 9.4 to 34.0 plus or minus 5.6, function score improved from 21.2 plus or minus 9.7 to 45.1 plus or minus 4.0, and alignment score improved from 6.0 plus or minus 2.8 to 9.8 plus or minus 0.9. Based on the Ankle Osteoarthritis Scale, the score for pain at its worst improved from a mean of 6.1 plus or minus 3.3 to 2.0 plus or minus 1.7. At final follow-up, ankle inversion stress radiography showed a talar tilting angle of 5.0° plus or minus 3.6° and an anterior drawer distance of 1.4 plus or minus 0.5 mm. Dislocation and migration of the implant were not observed.[22]

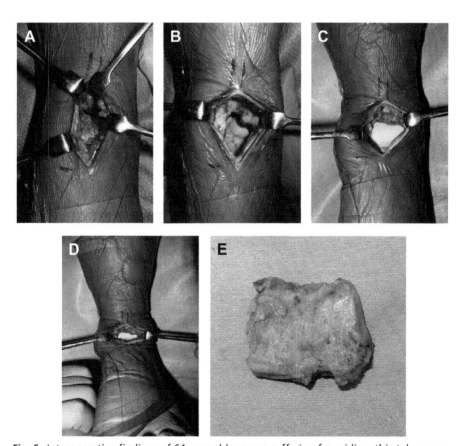

Fig. 6. Intraoperative findings of 64 year-old woman suffering from idiopathic talar necrosis. (*A*) The talar dome is collapsed and joint surface is widely degenerated. (*B*) The talus is completely removed. Artificial talar implant is inserted. (*C*) Plantar flexed position. (*D*) Dorsal flexed position. (*E*) Excised specimen. Talar dome is severely compressed and trabecula in the talar body has completely disappeared.

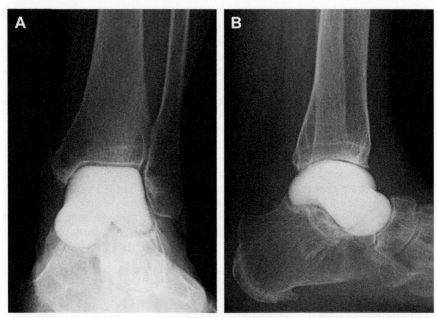

Fig. 7. Postoperative weightbearing radiography. (*A*) Anteroposterior view. (*B*) Lateral view.

In summary, the talus is surrounded by the tibia, fibula, calcaneus, and navicular, composing some joints in between with these bones. Customized alumina ceramic total talar prosthesis is an ideal implant for the treatment of severe talar osteonecrosis.

REFERENCES

1. Sanders RW, Lindvall E. Fractures and fracture-dislocation of the talus. In: Coughlin MJ, Mann RA, Saltzman CL, editors. Surgery of the foot and ankle. 8th edition. Philadelphia: Mosby Elsevier; 2007. p. 2074–136.
2. Gelberman RH, Mortensen WW. The arterial anatomy of the talus. Foot Ankle 1983;4:64–72.
3. Vallier HA, Nork SE, Barei DP, et al. Talar neck fractures: results and outcomes. J Bone Joint Surg Am 2004;86-A:1616–24.
4. Lindvall E, Haidukewych G, DiPasquale T, et al. Open reduction and stable fixation of isolated, displaced talar neck and body fractures. J Bone Joint Surg Am 2004;86-A:2229–37.
5. Adleberg JS, Smith GH. Corticosteroid-induced avascular necrosis of the talus. J Foot Surg 1991;30:66–9.
6. Harris RD, Silver RA. Atraumatic aseptic necrosis of the talus. Radiology 1973; 106:81–3.
7. Baron M, Paltiel H, Lander P, et al. Aseptic necrosis of the talus and calcaneal insufficiency fractures in a patient with pancreatitis, subcutaneous fat necrosis, and arthritis. Arthritis Rheum 1984;27:1309–13.
8. Macnicol MF, Ludlam CA. Does avascular necrosis cause collapse of the dome of the talus in severe haemophilia? Haemophilia 1999;5:139–42.
9. Kemnitz S, Moens P, Peerlinck K, et al. Avascular necrosis of the talus in children with haemophilia. J Pediatr Orthop B 2002;11:73–8.

10. Hong N, Du XK. Avascular necrosis of bone in severe acute respiratory syndrome. Clin Radiol 2004;59:602–8.
11. DiGiovanni CW, Patel A, Calfee R, et al. Osteonecrosis in the foot. J Am Acad Orthop Surg 2007;15:208–17.
12. Delanois RE, Mont MA, Yoon TR, et al. Atraumatic osteonecrosis of the talus. J Bone Joint Surg Am 1998;80-A:529–36.
13. Blair H. Comminuted fractures and fracture dislocation of the body of the astragalus. Am J Surg 1943;59:37.
14. Lionberger DR, Bishop JO, Tullos HS. The modified Blair fusion. Foot Ankle 1982; 3:60–2.
15. Tanaka Y, Takakura Y, Kadono K, et al. Alumina ceramic talar body prosthesis for idiopathic aseptic necrosis of the talus. Bioceramic 2002;15:805–8.
16. Kadono K, Tanaka Y, Sugimoto K, et al. Replacement of the body of the talus with alumina ceramic prosthesis for idiopathic aseptic necrosis. Orthop Ceramic Implant 2002;21:77–81 [in Japanese].
17. Ficat RP, Arlet J. Ischemia and necrosis of bone. Baltimore (MD): Wiliams and Wilkins; 1980. p. 171–82.
18. Mont MA, Schon LC, Hungerford MW, et al. Avascular necrosis of the talus treated by core decompression. J Bone Joint Surg Am 1996;78-B:827–30.
19. Pearce DH, Mongiardi CN, Fornasier VL, et al. Avascular necrosis of the talus: a pictorial essay. Radiographics 2005;25:399–410.
20. Shafa MH, Fernandez-Ulloa M, Rost RC, et al. Diagnosis of aseptic necrosis of the talus by bone scintigraphy. Clin Nucl Med 1983;8:50–3.
21. Horst F, Gilbert BJ, Nunley JA. Avascular necrosis of the talus: current treatment options. Foot Ankle Clin N Am 2004;9:757–73.
22. Taniguchi A, Takakura Y, Tanaka Y, et al. An alumina ceramic total talar prosthesis for osteonecrosis of the talus. J Bone Joint Surg Am 2015;97-A:1348–53.

Moving?

Make sure your subscription moves with you!

To notify us of your new address, find your **Clinics Account Number** (located on your mailing label above your name), and contact customer service at:

Email: journalscustomerservice-usa@elsevier.com

800-654-2452 (subscribers in the U.S. & Canada)
314-447-8871 (subscribers outside of the U.S. & Canada)

Fax number: 314-447-8029

Elsevier Health Sciences Division
Subscription Customer Service
3251 Riverport Lane
Maryland Heights, MO 63043

*To ensure uninterrupted delivery of your subscription, please notify us at least 4 weeks in advance of move.

Printed and bound by CPI Group (UK) Ltd, Croydon, CR0 4YY

08/05/2025

01864743-0002